The American Civil War Medical Series

Ira M. Rutkow, M.D., Dr.P.H.

1. John Ordronaux. *Hints on the Preservation of Health in Armies*. New York: 1861. BOUND WITH: Ordronaux. *Manual of Instructions for Military Surgeons*. New York: 1863.
2. Joseph Janvier Woodward. *The Hospital Steward's Manual*. Philadelphia: 1862.
3. Frank Hastings Hamilton. *A Practical Treatise on Fractures and Dislocations*. Philadelphia: 1860.
4. Francis Peyre Porcher. *Resources of the Southern Fields and Forests, Medical, Economical, and Agricultural*. Richmond: 1863.
5. William Alexander Hammond. *A Treatise on Hygiene*. Philadelphia: 1863.
6. Roberts Bartholow. *A Manual of Instructions for Enlisting and Discharging Soldiers*. Philadelphia: 1863.
7. Claude Bernard and Charles Huette. *Illustrated Manual of Operative Surgery and Surgical Anatomy*. Edited, with notes and additions . . . by William H. Van Buren and Charles E. Isaacs. New York: 1861.
8. Samuel Preston Moore. *Regulations of the C.S.A. Medical Department* IN: *Regulations for the Army of the Confederate States*. Richmond: 1862.
9. Charles Ravenscroft Greenleaf. *A Manual for the Medical Officers of the United States Army*. Philadelphia: 1864.
10. William Grace. *The Army Surgeon's Manual*. New York: 1864.
11. Joseph Janvier Woodward. *Outlines of the Chief Camp Diseases of the United States Armies*. Philadelphia: 1863.
12. *Confederate States Medical and Surgical Journal*. Richmond: January 1864 – February 1865.

HINTS ON THE PRESERVATION OF HEALTH IN ARMIES

AND

MANUAL OF INSTRUCTIONS FOR MILITARY SURGEONS

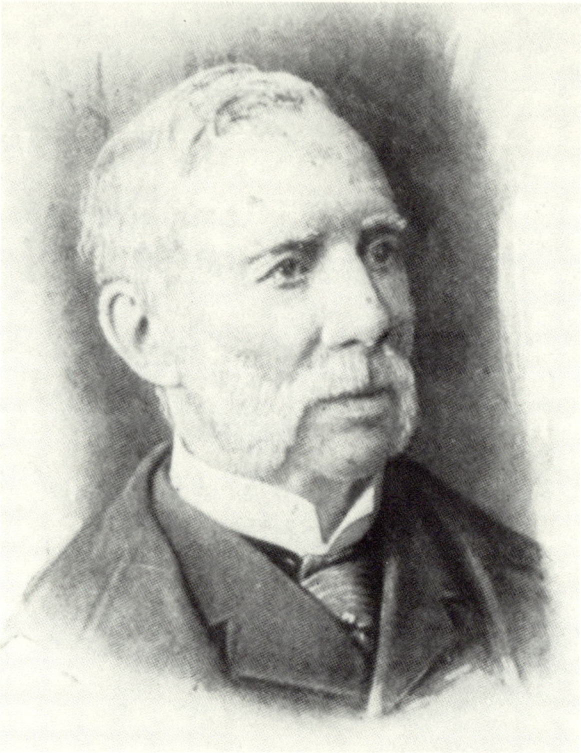

John Ordronaux
1830–1908

HINTS ON THE PRESERVATION OF HEALTH IN ARMIES

For the Use of Volunteer Officers and Soldiers

BOUND WITH

MANUAL OF INSTRUCTIONS FOR MILITARY SURGEONS

On the Examination of Recruits and Discharge of Soldiers

by John Ordronaux, M.D.

Reprinted with a Biographical Introduction

by Ira M. Rutkow, M.D., Dr.P.H.

Norman Publishing
San Francisco
1990

Published by Norman Publishing
720 Market Street
San Francisco, California 94102–2502

Library of Congress Cataloging-in-Publication Data

Ordronaux, John, 1830–1908.
Hints on the preservation of health in armies: bound with Manual of instructions for military surgeons.
p. cm. — (The American Civil War medical series : no. 1)
Reprint (1st work). Originally published: New York : Appleton, 1861. Reprint (2nd work). Originally published: New York : Van Nostrand, 1863.
ISBN 0–930405–34–X (alk. paper)
1. Military hygiene—Handbooks, manuals. etc. 2. United States—Armed Forces—Sanitary affairs—Handbooks, manuals, etc. 3. United States—Armed Forces—Medical examinations—handbooks, manuals, etc. 4. United States —Armed Forces—Recruiting, enlistment, etc.—Civil War, 1861–1865—Handbooks, Manuals, etc. 5. United States —History—Civil War, 1861–1865—Health aspects—Handbooks, manuals, etc. 6. Military Hygiene. 7. Military Medicine. I. Ordronaux, John, 1830–1908. Manual of instructions for military surgeons. II. Title. III. Series.
[DNLM: UH 065h 1861/63a]
UH623.0663 1991
617. 9′9—dc20
DNLM/DLC
for Library of Congress 90–14290
CIP

The American Civil War Medical Series, No. 1

This volume was reproduced from the original editions loaned from the Francis A. Countway Library of Medicine, Boston.

This book is printed on acid-free paper, and its binding materials have been chosen for strength and durability.

Manufactured in the United States of America.

John Ordronaux

John Ordronaux was born in New York City on August 3, 1830, the only son of John and Elizabeth Charreton Ordronaux. His father was a native of France but commanded the American privateer *Prince of Neufchatel* during the War of 1812. Unfortunately, Ordronaux's father died when he was only eleven years old. There is little mention made of his mother. However, it is known that the young man was subsequently adopted by John Moulton of Roslyn, Long Island. Ordronaux continued living with the Moultons until their deaths several years later. Their property was eventually acquired by William Cullen Bryant (1794–1878), with whom Ordronaux became quite friendly.

Ordronaux received traditional college preparatory training in New York City. He graduated from Dartmouth College in 1850 and Harvard Law School in 1852. For two years he practiced law in Taunton, Massachusetts, but soon resettled in his native city. In his leisure time Ordronaux began to study medicine under various private practitioners and attended numerous lecture sessions. Although he never received a formal M.D., he was awarded an honorary degree from the National Medical College (then the medical department of Columbian, now George Washington, University), Washington, D.C., in 1859. It was in this institution that he spent the following year as a lecturer on medical jurisprudence.

It was never Ordronaux's intention to enter the active practice of clinical medicine. Consequently, in 1860, he accepted an appointment as lecturer on medical jurisprudence in the law school of Columbia University in New York. The following year he was promoted to full professorial rank. With the outbreak of the Civil War he was made examining surgeon for volunteers in Brooklyn. In 1864 Ordronaux was appointed assistant surgeon of the Fifteenth Regiment of the National Guard of the State of New York. Although he never had any actual battlefield experience, Ordronaux utilized his medical service as background for his writings on military medicine.

With the end of the hostilities, Ordronaux continued his responsibilities at Columbia, remaining there until 1897. It was in medical jurisprudence that he became most widely known. For forty–eight years he was professor of this subject in various prominent schools of law and medicine. Among his other teaching positions were the chairs of medical jurisprudence at the University of Vermont School of Medicine (1865–73), Boston University Law School (1872–89), and Dartmouth Medical School (1873–1908).

In addition to his legal expertise, Ordronaux is considered among the leading alienists of late nineteenth-century America. *Alienist* is an obsolete term that was used to describe a physician who treated mental disorders. As a result of his expertise in law and the treatment of the mentally ill, Ordronaux served as the first New York state commissioner on lunacy from 1873 to 1882. During that time he revised the existing state lunacy laws. As a preeminent alienist he was often called to be a witness at many important criminal trials.

Ordronaux was a remarkably prolific author. It was during his initial military experience that he wrote his first major text *Hints on the Preservation of Health in Armies; For the Use of Volunteer Officers and Soldiers* (1861). A second edition with slight revisions came out two years later. This work is important because it is the first American book on military hygiene. Ordronaux was firm in his belief that precautionary measures needed to be taken to protect troops against diseases that were often preventable.

Ordronaux's other major medical book is the *Manual of Instructions for Military Surgeons; On the Examinations of Recruits and Discharge of Soldiers* (1863). The *Manual* was prepared at the request of the United States Sanitary Commission. Ordronaux states in the preface that his book is "for the most part, a free translation of the French code" of instruction on the subjects of the enlistment and discharge of soldiers. The French code of 1862 details diseases of over thirty-five organs and regions of the body. With the information contained in the *Manual*, the military physician was able to complete an examination of a new recruit in a more orderly fashion. Most importantly, it helped the examining doctor deter any attempts at malingering.

Among Ordronaux's important legal works are

the *Report to the United States Sanitary Commission on a System for the Economical Relief of Disabled Soldiers, and on Certain Proposed Amendments to Our Present Pension Laws* (1864); *The Jurisprudence of Medicine in Its Relations to the Law of Contracts, Torts, and Evidence, with a Supplement on the Liabilities of Vendors of Drugs* (1869); *Commentaries on the Lunacy Laws of New York and on the Judicial Aspects of Insanity in Common Law and in Equity, Including Procedure, as Expounded in England and the United States* (1878); *The Plea of Insanity as an Answer to Indictment* (1880); *Judicial Problems Relating to the Disposal of Insane Criminals* (1881); and *Constitutional Legislation in the United States* (1891). Although Ordronaux's reputation as a practicing lawyer was not well known, his peers regarded him as a keen intellect. Consequently, he was frequently employed to write legal briefs for many of his fellow professionals.

Ordronaux was a lifelong bachelor. Described as a small, slender, frail-looking man, he was said to be sensitive to even the slightest bit of physical hostility. Quiet, unassuming, and socially withdrawn, Ordronaux lived for many years with a widow and her family in Roslyn. Although a man of ample financial resources, he was not self-indulgent and denied himself many material possessions. He was subject to frequent bouts of depression that were attributed in part to his never having had a real home, stable adolescence, or family. Never one to participate in the politics of organized medicine, Ordronaux spent most of his spare time in intellectual pursuits. Most notable was his poetic translation of the *Regimen Sanitatis Salernitanum*: *Code of Health of the School of Salernum* (1870). He also translated Horace from the Greek.

Ordronaux received the honorary degree of LL.D. from Trinity College in Connecticut in

1870 and the same degree from Dartmouth College in 1895. He was a member of the Episcopalian church, which he attended on a regular basis, and occasionally acted as a lay reader. On Sunday, January 19, 1908, Ordronaux suffered a cerebral hemorrhage. He became unconscious immediately and died the following morning in Roslyn. There were no living relatives at the time of his death.

HINTS

ON

THE PRESERVATION OF

HEALTH IN ARMIES.

FOR THE USE OF

VOLUNTEER OFFICERS AND SOLDIERS.

BY

JOHN ORDRONAUX, M. D.,

PROFESSOR OF MEDICAL JURISPRUDENCE IN COLUMBIA COLLEGE,

"It is surely the first duty of a Government, as well as of a commander, to adopt every possible precaution which can guarantee the health and life of the army, to which the honor and even the safety of the state are intrusted."—MACLEOD, *Surgery of the Crimean War.*

NEW YORK:

D. APPLETON AND COMPANY,

443 & 445 BROADWAY.

1861.

TO

WILLIAM CULLEN BRYANT,

AS A TESTIMONIAL OF RESPECT,

FROM HIS FRIEND AND NEIGHBOR,

THE AUTHOR.

PREFACE.

The Preservation of Health in Armies, is everywhere a subject of recognized importance. So much, in fact, depends upon it, that precautionary measures in this behalf can never be exaggerated. All that can be done, should be done to protect troops against preventable disease.

It seems to have been formerly believed, that the presence of a Surgeon in each regiment was all sufficient for this purpose; and that officers and men could go their way free from any responsibility or apprehension on that score. But experience has proved that the preservation of health, in either one man, or many, is not purely *objective* with Surgeons. Too much, in this particular, is expected from them, and too little is done by officers to coöperate with them. Armies, like patients, must act in concert with their medical advisers, and make the matter of health *subjective* as well as objective. Officers and men need an insight into the general principles of hygiene, in order to be able to assist, themselves, in furthering prophylactic measures.

To supply them with the requisite amount of information, the accompanying popular manual has therefore been prepared. In this, nothing like a formal treatise or text-book has been attempted. Its brevity, its omission of all scientific discussion, and of many statistical tables, will sufficiently indicate that the mission it is designed to perform is one eminently *suggestive*, and not in any sense *authoritative*. To "help, rather than to hinder," is the maxim which has guided me in its compilation; and desiring more especially to make this little "hornbook" of use to military officers and soldiers, rather than to Surgeons who possess such great textual authorities as Hamilton, Gross, Hennen, Larrey, and Boudin—I have consequently avoided as much as possible the terminology of medical science, as well as the discussion of medical principles.

Trusting that these desultory thoughts, which have thus crystallized themselves into the form of "Hints," may be productive of some measure of good, not only in provoking greater watchfulness over preventable disease; but also by stimulating other minds to worthier efforts in the cause of Military Hygiene, I now commit them to the hands of my countrymen, asking only to be permitted to remind them, that "Good fortune ever fights on the side of prudence."

J. O.

ROSLYN, near New York,
May 23, 1861.

CONTENTS.

CHAPTER		PAGE
I.—On Armies,	. . . . . .	9
II.—On the Medical Examination of Recruits,		17
III.—On the Education of Recruits,	. .	22
IV.—On the Construction and Hygiene of Barracks,	. . . . .	36
V.—On the March,	. . . . .	41
VI.—On the Camp,	. . . . . .	52
VII.—On the Food of Soldiers, and Education of Cooks,	. . . . . .	61
VIII.—On the Clothing,	. . . . .	76
IX.—On the Prevention of Disease in General, and the Individual Preservation of Health,	. . . . .	82
X.—On Hospitals,	. . . . . .	105
Appendix.—U. S. Army Ambulance Regulations, and Hospital Stores,	. . .	115

HINTS

ON THE

HEALTH OF ARMIES.

CHAPTER I.

ON ARMIES.

It may be stated as a fundamental maxim in the science of warfare, that *a state of perfect bodily health is indispensable to the successful discharge of a soldier's duties.* Whatever influence (whether of soil, climate, diet, or discipline) interrupts this physical condition, disqualifies him to that extent for active usefulness. Armies being aggregations of individuals, each contributing something towards the strength, support, and moral influence of the general mass, it follows that the withdrawal of any units from this sum is *pro tanto* a diminution of the effectiveness of the whole. And worse than this, the weak and sick, in proportion as their numbers increase, demoralize the healthy, as well by the spectacle of their infirmities as by the increased duties, responsibilities, and apprehensions for the future which must inevitably fall upon them. A sick army is always a demoralized force. Men, whose organic functions are either interrupted or vitiated by disease, can not perform their duties as before. They may still have courage, but courage in such cases becomes simply a spasm, and is lacking in all qualities of endurance. The first duty of a skilful commander is, therefore, to preserve the health of his troops; for their health like their ammunition is the instrument with which they can alone hope to conquer.

It seems to be hardly known outside of armies that the proportion of their mortality, under the most favorable circumstances, is *twice* that of civil life, although in this latter so many patent causes of disease manifest themselves as would make us infer differently. Dr. Farr, from observations made on the British army, presents us with the following fearful statistics:

Relation of Mortality.		Deaths annually to 1,000 living.
Ages.	Occupation.	Ratio.
20 to 25	Civilians.	8·4
	Soldiers,	17·0
25 to 30	Civilians,	9·2
	Soldiers,	18·3
30 to 35	Civilians,	10·2
	Soldiers,	18·4
35 to 40	Civilians,	11·6
	Soldiers,	19·2

That this mortality is reducible to a ratio at least equal to that of civil life, is not to be questioned; for we see it already so foreshadowed in the less percentage observable among old soldiers, who, without any additional safeguards to health beyond those possessed by their younger brethren, are yet from *habit* and induration protected from those lurking morbific agencies which decimate the latter; and if so reducible, then it is the duty of the state to prevent it, because preventable mortality is criminal mortality, and the responsibility for its occurrence rests at the door of those through whose negligence it has happened.

It is to a want of observance of simple hygienic rules, that we must charge this needless waste of human life; for it is not sufficient to say that the inevitable duties of a soldier—guard-mounting, drills, fatiguing marches, changes of climate, diet, and dwelling—necessitate so high a ratio of mortality. Experience, in fact, proves the contrary. Hunters and trappers are proverbially healthy men, although exposed to as great fatigues, hardship, extremes of weather, and vicissitudes of diet as soldiers. The cause of this excessive mortality is plainly due to something different from any one of the above assigned reasons, or even all of them combined.

Applied either separately or jointly to any one individual, they do not, as in the case of hunters, justify us in considering them as efficient causes. We must look, therefore, for another and more predisposing agency in the production of disease. And that agency we shall find in the *gregarious* mode of living, and the general negligence of preventive measures which prevails in most armies. The former is undoubtedly inevitable, but it need not be accompanied by a total disregard of those rules of health which are found indispensable to the well-being of all large communities. Men congregated in masses, and in small areas—overtasked, uncleanly, and improperly fed, whether they be soldiers or artisans, are subjected to precisely the same laws of health and disease, and the violation of those laws always entails the same fearful penalty upon all.

Military science has made stupendous progress within the present generation. In the improvement of arms in particular, it has signally triumphed. So terrible is its enginery now, that the possibility of any defence against its effects is almost abandoned. The art of offence has culminated. Before the destructive missiles hurled from the mouths of rifled cannon, neither wood nor stone can stand; and the reduction of any fortress against which such ordnance is brought to bear is simply a question of time. But with all the glory which the art of warfare has acquired, and with all the good it may have accomplished in equalizing disparity of forces, it will yet have failed in the first of all essentials, and left an unrelenting foe in its rear, so long as it ignores the necessity of incorporating within its principles a well-digested system of hygiene. Without this, the direst enemy will be found always in the very midst of the largest assemblage of men; striking right and left, at night and in the day, the "lean, cold hand of disease" will dismember an army more certainly than those who, heralded by drum and bugle, and visible to sight, fall on it only with bayonet and sabre-stroke. It was Frederic the Great who used to remark with a sigh, that fever annually robbed him of more men than seven pitched battles. And yet, long as this startling truth has been known, and fearfully as it has illustrated itself in every army since the day when it was first uttered, no adequate measures have yet been taken in many countries to prevent the evil which thus decimates their armies. Overcrowded, ill-ventilated barracks, small, foul tents, indifferent provisions, badly organized hospitals, will continue to do their work of silent destruction, until medical men are allowed some power and discretion in the housing, feeding, and superintendence of troops. When this shall be done, we can hope for a marked diminution in the ratio of their mortality; but until it is done, we must expect to see the flower of every army cut off, and the state shorn of its most useful members in times of direst necessity.

It is upon officers, therefore, of every grade, that rests the responsibility of preserving the health of their men. From the highest to the humblest each has his portion to command, and inasmuch as any wanton, unjustifiable waste of life, either in an assault or on a battle-field, exposes an officer to a court-martial, so with the same propriety, and by parity of reason, should any negligence of sanitary rules, resulting in unnecessary loss of life, expose him to the same penalties. With a sufficient medical staff at his elbow, it is idle for the officer to attempt to shield himself behind the plea of ignorance, or those petrified formalities which are the heir-looms of inflated officialism. In the presence of elementary forces hastening to develop disease, red-tape and official rubrics must vanish; hygiene, without waiting for the fecial college to declare war, must be allowed to attack the enemy and to demolish him, ere he has assembled his forces; after which "*general orders*" can again march on in their old conventional ways.

A chief source of disturbance to the health of all new levies is found in the *suddenness* with which they are translated from the comforts of home, and the moderate, generally self-imposed and self-regulated duties of civil life, to the extremes of diet, (quantity and quality,) fatigue and exposure, incidental to active operations in the field. This suddenness of transition is always depressing to the nervous energies in any contingency, either of civil or military life, but particularly, and more dangerously so in the latter, because of the necessary inability of obtaining periods of intervening rest during which nature can gradually recover herself from the direct and reflex shocks under whose influence she is laboring.* Placed in this po-

* The statistics of the French army show the following to be the average proportion of its mortality:—

	LOSS IN EACH 1,000.
During the 1st year of service,	7·5
" " 2d " "	6·5
" " 3d " "	5·2
" " 4th " "	4·3
" " 5th " "	3·
" " 6th " "	2·
" " 7th " "	2·

It is thus seen that the first year is the most fatal to soldiers.

sition, the soldier may be considered as directly inviting an attack of disease; nor will it be slow to appear, or fail to assume an epidemic character when corresponding in type to the constitutional tendencies of the season.

Now, the best protection to health is the possession of health, which like a shield protects us against morbific influences only so long as we preserve it entire. Other things being equal, in any exposure to the sources of disease a man in vigorous health will longest endure, while those of inferior physical tone soonest succumb. Hence, it becomes, in an economical point of view a matter of the gravest importance to the state, to see that its armies are formed out of the most able-bodied of its adult population. The soldier must be healthy at the start, if he would enter the service with any hope of being useful to his country, or to acquire distinction for himself. Statistics show that disease is nearly *four times* * more formidable to armies than bullets, and the weak are very sure to fall first beneath the shafts of this unerring marksman. This being the case, science is called upon to provide means adequate to interrupting all preventable diseases in the soldier when actually in the service, as also to sift out from among recruits all those whose physical constitution is per-

* The mortality tables in the British army in the Crimea show that in the first five months (from Sept. 6, 1854, to Feb. 5, 1855) it lost at the rate of 391 *per thousand* by disease, and only 108 by wounds. The French, in the last six months of the campaign, had of killed and wounded 21,937 to 101,128 sick with various diseases.

manently defective. We must have healthy, well-knit men for recruits in order to make strong and resolute soldiers, and we must have strong and resolute soldiers in order to form invincible armies.

It will be perceived from these observations, that a well ordained and enforced system of *hygiene* is indispensable to the maintenance of a healthy army; and in order that such a system may work to its greatest advantage, not only the surgeons who plan and direct its details, but, and as far as can be intelligible to non-medical men, all officers should know enough of its outlines to enable them the better to coöperate with their medical advisers.*

The first step in the formation of an army is the selection of young and able-bodied recruits. And for the purpose of securing these, a thorough medical examination of each candidate should be made. This examination must be conducted by the medical inspector in person, assisted by a non-commissioned officer, and always by daylight.

* The opposition to sanitary reforms, which is encountered not solely among the ignorant poor, but too often among educated laymen, leads to the belief that the cause of antagonism is similar in both classes, and resides in that *ignorance* of the powers of hygiene, which accepts disease as a *fate*, and consequently scoffs at those who endeavor to avert its shafts. When men can be made to believe that health is our natural state, and that God has given us means for preserving it in the very elements around us, they will no longer hesitate as to the line of their duty, but will zealously coöperate in all efforts to prevent disease.

CHAPTER II.

GENERAL RULES FOR THE EXAMINATION OF RECRUITS.

THE surgeon, having first satisfied himself that the candidate is within the prescribed age, (18 to 45,) will order him to be stripped naked, and placed with his back to the light.

GENERAL ANATOMICAL FEATURES.—Placing himself at a convenient distance he will first scan the anatomical proportions, or general conformation of body, shape of the head, chest, abdomen, and limbs of the recruit, viewing him in front, rear, and sidewise; after which he will command him to march forward and backward, cause him to bend forward, jump, kneel, sit and rise rapidly, all the while noticing whether there be free and unembarrassed motion of the large joints and muscles.

FIRST OBSERVATION.—The surgeon will now proceed to a particular examination of the *head*, *ears*, *the hearing*, *eyes*, and *teeth*. The eyes, and their power of sight require the closest scrutiny. For this purpose the recruit should be tested with suitable objects at various distances. Each eye should be separately tested as by taking aim, &c.; tests for color blindness should also be applied.

Second Observation.—Examinations must then be made of the *neck*, *chest*, (*external* and by *auscultation*,) *back* and *loins*, including the *arms*, their flexor and extensor muscles, the *hands* and all the digital muscles, and particularly all the articulations. Every finger, the wrists, the elbow and shoulder joints must be flexed and extended, separately and together.

Third Observation.—The abdomen and buttocks, the testicles, scrotum, and inguinal regions, the penis, and anus must next be inspected.

Fourth Observation.—The *thighs* and *calves* of the legs, with all their articulations, must be inspected; varicose veins must not be overlooked.

Fifth Observation.—The feet and their shape; the toes, their joints and muscles, must be carefully inspected. Also the mode of step. Is the recruit *splay-footed?* Do the toes turn in or out?

Sixth Observation.—The *stature* of the recruit should now be measured, and where there is any suspicion of his attempt to increase its appearance, he should be measured supine, instead of erect. It should be noticed also whether he has had the small-pox or been vaccinated.*

* Vaccination, although not insisted upon as a prerequisite to enlistment, should be performed upon all who have not been thus protected, as soon as they reach a depot. The vesicle will not prevent the use of the arm in drilling, and is too slight an in-

DISQUALIFYING DISEASES.

These may be divided into two classes, viz.: such as imply *absolute*, and such as imply *relative* incapacity for military service.

CLASS FIRST.

Relating to Organic or Articular Degeneration, General Mal-conformation or Absence of Parts.

Phthisis, aneurism of large arteries, scrofulous ulcers, voluminous goitre; privation of sight or hearing; dumbness; permanent aphonia; loss of an arm, leg, foot, hand; curvature of the long bones; rickets; anchylosis; paralysis, or retraction of the flexor or extensor muscles of a limb; atrophy; obesity; talipes.

CLASS SECOND.

Relating to Particular Affections of the Head, Trunk, Limbs, and Skin.

HEAD.

Extensive injuries of skull, (depression, exfoliation,) giving rise to occasional giddiness, drowsiness, pains in the head, and affections of the intellect; loss of right eye; fistula lachrymalis; habitual diseases of eyes, ophthalmia, rheums, &c.; weakness of sight; myopia; nyctalopia; amblyopia; deformity of nose,

convenience to be thought of as against the advantages secured. Let this duty to society never be omitted by surgeons.

capable of interrupting freedom of respiration; ozæna; caries and incurable polypus; incurably fetid breath; discharges from the ears; loss of upper or lower incisors; necrosis of jaw; fistulas of the maxillary sinuses or salivary glands; difficulty of deglutition, from paralysis or other incurable lesion; chronic affections of the organs of hearing, voice, or speech, sensiby impairing their use.

NECK, CHEST, ARMS, HANDS.

Ulcers, and scrofulous tumors; deformity of chest; Pott's disease, or any spinal curvature affecting respiration or the carrying of arms and wearing of accoutrements; phthisis, (incipient;) chronic asthma; habitual hæmoptysis; total loss of the thumb or of the fore-finger of the right hand, or two other fingers of one hand, or the mutilation of the last joints of one or several fingers of the *right* hand; * paralysis of either arm; affections of any muscles or joints in the arm or hand impeding their free motion, (arthritis, chronic rheumatism,) and incurable deformities in any of these parts.

ABDOMEN.

Irreducible hernias; calculus; gravel; habitual incontinence or retention of urine; fistulas and se-

* These deformities do not disqualify the recruit for service *absolutely*, as he may still discharge the duties of a *miner*, *sapper*, *pioneer*, or *artillerist*—and many others above enumerated would still leave him in a condition to perform certain *garrison* duties. The disqualifying diseases which we have cited, refer more particularly to recruits designed for *active* service in the field.

vere diseases of the urinary passages; strangulation of testicle, sarcocele; hydrocele; varicocele; and all incurable affections of the scrotum, testicles, penis, or spermatic cord; ulcerated hæmorrhoids; fistula in ano; periodical hæmorrhoidal flux; *habitual* incontinence of fæces, and prolapsus ani; chronic weakness of the loins, accompanied by inveterate lumbago.

LOWER LIMBS AND FEET.

Large varices; incurable ulcers; affections of muscles or joints impeding their free motion. Severe diseases of the bones; loss of great toe, or two toes of a foot; incurable deformities of feet.

SKIN AND CONSTITUTIONAL AFFECTIONS.

All contagious diseases when become chronic and inveterate, such as tinea, herpes, psora, elephantiasis and lepra; well-marked cachexy of a scorbutic or glandular character; debility and extreme emaciation; a too diminutive or tall stature accompanied by weakness, and leanness or obesity; gout and sciatica; chronic rheumatism impeding the free motion of the trunk or limbs; epilepsy; convulsions; chorea; general or partial paralysis; imbecility.

NOTE.—The surgeon will, on a printed blank furnished for this purpose, note the *cause* of rejection of every recruit.

CHAPTER III.

EDUCATION OF RECRUITS.

Recruits, when assembled and about to be drafted into various corps, should first of all things be *classified* with reference to such antecedents of trade or vocation, or such bodily or mental capacity as can impart to them predominant qualifications for the different arms of the service. By this means much time will be gained which otherwise would have to be consumed in a species of rough and hasty apprenticeship in these several preliminaries to military usefulness. This apprenticeship is always more or less chafing to young recruits, who are apt to suppose that once enlisted they are fit to undertake all a soldier's duties, and who repudiate every idea of mechanical handicraft as incompatible with a military profession. Yet learn they must, and the more nearly the duty corresponds to former avocations, the more rapidly they will learn, and the more easily and cheerfully they will labor. Time and health will thus both be economized.

The following table will illustrate the subject by

furnishing the elements on which such classifications should be based.

CLASSIFICATIONS BASED ON ANTECEDENT QUALIFICATIONS.*

Corps.	Adjuvant qualifications.
Engineer.	Should have worked in a furnace or forge, been a blacksmith, nailsmith, cartwright, carpenter, joiner, miner, mason, bridge-builder, cooper, boat-builder, saddler or harness-maker, and generally acquainted with tools.
Artillery.	Should have been a cartwright, carman, or worked in iron and wood; accustomed to ride, drive, or tend horses.
Cavalry.	Should have been accustomed to riding, driving, or tending horses. Should be tall and large-framed.
Riflemen.	Should be lithe, well-knit, not over-tall, muscular, accustomed to long tramps, to hunting, and to the use of fire-arms.
Infantry of the line.	Same as foregoing, except being taller and larger-framed.

* The *dynamometer* is an instrument whose assistance should be invoked in classifying men for service in those branches requiring great *manual* or *renal* strength. In selecting artillerists, whether on sea or land, sappers and miners, and others of kindred occupations, its scale should always be applied, in order to determine the positive power possessed. We accordingly subjoin

In the European service *stature* is a prominent element of classification. It is not so yet with us. Extremes only are avoided.

As raw troops are an unreliable material with which to undertake a campaign, serving too often only to encumber hospitals and to confuse the movements of regulars in times of peril, it becomes of the greatest importance to give the recruit the benefit of some probationary exercises in barracks by way of weaning him from old habits, and gradually strengthening and disciplining him for the severe duties of the field. As this discipline involves a radical change in diet, exercise, sleep, and clothing, it is necessary that it should be conducted under the immediate direction

a table illustrative of the averages of human strength as measured by it, in the French service.

RENAL STRENGTH.				MANUAL STRENGTH.							
Age.	Power.	Age.	Power.	Age.	With both hands.	With Right.	With Left.	Age.	With both hands.	With Right.	With Left.
	Myr.		Myr.		Kilo.				Kilo.		
11	4.8	19	13.2	11	29.2	10.7	9.2	19	79.4	35.4	35.0
12	5.1	20	13.8	12	33.6	13.9	11.7	20	84.3	39.3	37.1
13	6.9	21	14.6	13	39.8	16.6	15.0	21	86.4	43.0	38.0
14	8.1	25	15.6	14	47.9	21.4	18.8	25	88.7	44.1	40.0
15	8.8	30	15.4	15	57.1	27.8	22.6	30	89.0	44.7	41.3
16	10.2	40	12.2	16	63.9	32.3	26.8	40	87.0	41.2	38.3
17	12.6	50	10.1	17	71.0	36.2	31.9	50	74.0	36.4	33.0
18	13.0	60	9.3	18	79.2	38.6	35.0	60	56.0	30.3	26.0

See *Dictionnaire des Sciences Medicales*, art. *Dynamometre*.

The French Kilogramme is equal to 2 lbs. 3 oz. 5 drs. Avoirdupois.

The French Myriagramme is equal to *ten* Kilogrammes.

of a medical officer, in order that the constitutional idiosyncrasies of some may be duly and gradually overcome, instead of being rudely shocked by an unrelaxing severity which may tend to develop disease otherwise preventable. The medical officer, therefore, should be allowed to grant dispensations to recruits newly enlisted, from the performance of certain duties, or in the duration of their execution, until satisfied that the recruit is able to bear them. Thus guard-mounting after the fatigues of the day should be regulated in duration according to the ability of the recruit, the season, and the weather; exercise of a new kind to him should be similarly conducted, the idea always being to *convert* the recruit into a soldier by making every step of the apprenticeship a profitable one in health and a stimulus to his ambition, instead of breaking him down by the first week's discipline, and keeping him in hospital for a month to get over it.

That exercise in the open air invigorates the frame all from experience know. By increasing the activity of our functions, and rendering us less susceptible to the influences of weather, it enables us to perform fatiguing labors without any ill consequences, and thus develops in all a high measure of muscular ability. But this result is not immediately to be attained, any more than the growth of the body can be compelled beyond nature's own ordained periods. Muscle like mind must be gradually educated, and in both undue tension or ill-regulated effort only serves to retard development. A certain time is required to habituate the frame to *continuous* effort of even the most moderate kind, and the longer the period of apprenticeship, the more confirmed will be its good effects. Among the Romans, military education began in extreme youth. Gymnastics and games of all kinds inured the citizen from early life to the fatigues of field exercises. Hence, when he arrived at man's estate he was a perfected soldier in physical development already.

But with us, no preliminary education of the muscles in youth prepares the recruit for the active duties of the soldier. Fresh from the long-debilitating life of the counting-room, the factory, or the thousand sedentary pursuits of the civilian, he steps into the ranks of the army, and loads himself down with arms and baggage to make a fatiguing march of many miles. Weak in his shoulders, his loins, his wrists, and his knees—not carrying so much weight once in a year as his knapsack amounts to, and hardly ever marching off ten consecutive miles at any one time or sleeping out of his own bed, it is little short of cruelty to take such a man into the field and impose all its unrelenting hardships upon him. His life is jeopardized from the very start by his own insufficiency of muscular discipline, and he can hardly be of use to the state although burning with the ardor of patriotism.

Let officers, then, remember that the human machine is capable of performing only a very limited amount of any new duty at first, and that if pushed beyond this, its energies are exhausted and a typhoid state supervenes. Dr. Levy, one of the surgeons in chief to the French army, remarks that forced marches, heavy drills, and too prolonged exercises always increase the hospital list; and even where the muscular strain is not sufficient to produce acute disease, and yet daily transcends the measure of individual strength and organic repair, however slightly, it gradually and insidiously produces a state of deterioration and general debility.

In order to avoid so disastrous a result, the rule of exercise should be one of *gradual progression.* It is always better to stop short of actual fatigue. For this purpose, recruits should be drilled with moderation at first. Twice daily, with intervening hours of rest, the drill not extending beyond *two* hours at each session, seems about as much as any new recruit coming from sedentary pursuits can endure. This amount can be increased, of course, after a few days' practice with the majority of men; but there will always be some who will lag under the effort, and to these, hygiene, rather than severity, had better be applied. Muscular vigor is not a fixed and definite power in man. It varies with the age, original constitution, diet, profession, season, and weather. These elements must be fully considered and have due weight allowed them, when allotting measures of exercise and effort to recruits. By degrees, all may be brought to bear the amount of exercise required by the most laborious kinds of drilling, but caution at the outset must be observed with the *younger* recruits. A month is a short time in which to make a penman, with attenuated wrists and fingers, capable of twirling a musket or sword; or a tailor or shoemaker with shrunken legs capable of marching fifteen miles, day after day, fully armed and equipped. Some may attain to this ability in that time, but it is certain that all can not. The competent should speedily be transferred to their various places in the field, and the tardy kept drilling until in like manner perfected. This graduation of the former will serve greatly to stimulate the latter.

Another fact to be borne in mind is, that all exercises do not produce the same effects upon the system. Some develop one class of muscles, and some another. Steady, measured exercise which produces a harmonious development of all the muscles, rather than strong, violent efforts which develop only particular parts, is what the soldier needs. In modern times, it is not athletes capable of bending the bow of Ulysses, or wielding the club of Hercules, that we need, but active, lithe, symmetrical, and indurated men. The French zouave or chasseur is not a Hercules in size or even strength, but like a combination of steel and whalebone, he wears well under fatigue, and springs back from it with wonderful recuperation.

Most authorities in military surgery are agreed in denouncing the enlistment of men *under* 20 years of age. Statistics show that enlistments made in violation of this suggestion only serve to encumber the hospitals, without otherwise increasing the strength of armies. As an illustration of the importance of *age*, it is only sufficient to state that, in the French campaign of 1805, the army marched some 1,200 miles to reach the battle-field of Austerlitz, without meeting with any appreciable sickness or loss in numbers. Its youngest soldiers were 22 years old, and had served *two* years. But in the campaign of 1809 the army marched only a short distance from Germany into Austria, and yet, before reaching Vienna, all its hospitals were filled. The majority of its new conscripts were under *twenty* years of age. It was on this occasion that Napoleon wrote to the legislative senate asking for a new levy, and saying: "*I must have grown men; boys serve only to encumber the hospitals and roadsides.*"

Recruits should first be drilled in the lightest of their usual garbs, (fatigue dress.) No overcoat or knapsacks should be worn until fully accustomed to the manual of arms. Afterwards these *impedimenta*, as the Romans called baggage, can be put on *gradually*. The drill over, the men should be ordered to wash their faces, hands, and arms, if the weather be warm, otherwise it is not necessary. These precautionary measures will both refresh them, as well as afford protection against imprudence in drinking cold water when overheated, and in exposure to draughts of air. It should never be omitted in summer.

Recruits should not be exercised *fasting*, nor in the full blaze of a noon-day sun in summer, and it is well to allow during the drill an occasional intermission for a few minutes for the purposes of rest. In order to guard them against the effects of the ever-repeated imprudence of unbuttoning their jackets after drilling to "cool off," the last part of the exercise should be reduced in vigor, and thus afford the circulation an opportunity gradually to diminish its rapidity.

The new exercise of prolonged running, better known as the "gymnastic step," is one of exceeding danger when performed with knapsack and accoutrements. The very constrained condition of the chest, particularly when a cross-belt is worn, impedes free respiration; the lungs are rapidly inflated, but only in their upper portion, while the lower lobes retain too long the air required to keep them dilated; whence follow an increasing engorgement and difficulty of respiration, verging almost towards suffocation. Great care is consequently required in initiating soldiers into this most trying of all exercises, for an error in excess here may speedily cause hæmorrhage, and permanent pulmonary or cardiac mischief. The first thing to be taught the soldier is to harmonize the breathing with the motions of the limbs. This act once acquired, he can run, even when burdened, with facility.

But there will always be found a large number of men who cannot run with facility. These will ever lag in such an exercise, and so interrupt the order of the column. Where special duties of running devolve upon any corps, it would be proper to recruit it from among those who are possessed of this faculty. As a general rule, small, lithe men, with broad shoulders, run and march best, and it is also to be observed that, past the age of forty, few men can follow this rapid step. Zouaves and riflemen, therefore, should be formed out of only young men.

Horsemanship is another of those exercises which require gradual progression. Although unquestionably healthy for the majority of men, there are yet those in whom ill consequences follow from its excessive practice. Hernias, and inflammations of the testicles often testify to the effects of incessant jolting in the saddle, and it is advisable for all horsemen to protect themselves against these accidents by wearing a suspensory bandage.

But the best exercises for the soldier are those in which he does not simply obey a command mechanically, but employs his own mind and body under the varying impulse of each present necessity. Thus in *fencing*, *broadsword* and *bayonet* exercise, he has to exert his own faculties of offence and defence, independent of the command of any superior; and the necessary extension of limbs, variety of attitudes, and rapidity of motion which it requires—the sudden contraction and relaxation of muscle, and the acceleration of respiration which it occasions, heightens the tone of the whole system. The eyesight is quickened, the chest enlarged, the joints strengthened, the body rendered supple and muscular so as to secure the best and readiest use of all its faculties. No one, who has seen the almost miraculous change in the port and strength of the soldier, which can be wrought by fencing and the bayonet exercise, will hesitate to assign them the first rank in the hygiene of a military education.

Between the hours of drill, the men should, under the guidance of their various officers, be taught how to clean and keep in repair their arms; how to make cartridges; fill shells; take apart and pack gun-carriages; make fuzes gabions fascines, &c. Any little occupation like this, by keeping the mind active, stimulates it to acquisition and raises the soldier's own self-respect.

Besides the drill within the barrack-yard, and as part of the same in time consumed, recruits should be made to perform daily marches in the field, fully equipped. They should begin with short distances, then longer ones, throwing out flanking parties and advanced guards, establishing pickets, encamping and striking tents while on the march. The art of throwing up intrenchments, making and repelling feigned attacks, should also be taught, in order to inspire them with confidence and self-reliance. These daily marches varying in direction, length, and duties performed, would preserve the spirits as well as the health of the recruit, and give him what he so much thirsts for—a practical idea of the contingencies of war.

In addition to the moral effect of keeping soldiers actively employed, the gymnastic discipline derived from marching each day in different directions—from digging, lifting, running, leaping—in hardening the muscles and developing the strength of the soldier, is the very best school in which to perfect his attainments. Nothing but gymnastic exercises made the light-armed Greeks so terrible in battle; and nothing but similar exercises have made that perfection of all modern soldiers, the French zouave. And, inasmuch as these field exercises are the very ones which the soldier is eventually brought to perform in war, he cannot be too well prepared for them during the period of his military pupilage.

Habits of cleanliness should be particularly insisted upon wherever practicable. Soap, towels, and brushes can always be used in barracks, and every morning each man should be made to wash *face*, *neck*, *arms*, and *feet* in cold water. At roll-call, each corporal should report the state of his squad in this particular, to the officer in command.

As much of the *outside* clothing as can be dispensed with should be removed at night. This should be *insisted* upon, and the men, instead of one blanket, should be furnished with *two*, to compensate for the deficiency in covering thus created. In the field, when the soldier cannot undress, *one* blanket *may* be sufficient,* but this one should be of the firmest texture; and, as a further protection in wet weather, a rubber blanket should be given him.

Owing to the porous nature of all textile fabrics, and their retention of organic matter in the form of emanations, blankets should be daily aired and ex-

* The Government furnishes each man with only *one* blanket, and that often as *sleasy*, almost, as a bolting-cloth. This criminal neglect of health should be palliated by giving the soldier a *rubber* blanket in addition, thus keeping him *dry*, if not warm.

posed to the sunlight. If the weather will not admit of its being done out of doors, it should be done indoors, and in rooms with open fire-places and lighted fires. At least once a week, every well man should be compelled to *thoroughly* wash himself and change his body clothing.

The proper ventilation of dormitories at night, and of guard-rooms during the day, must never be overlooked, and recruits should be taught the importance of appreciating and enforcing rules for its observance.

Corporals should also make an inspection of the men when in bed, to see that they are properly undressed, that their garments are dry, and that the orders of the medical officer, relating to the wearing of particular articles of clothing, are strictly observed.

Wherever practicable, daily bathing in summer should be permitted and advised. But it should be done under the eye of an officer, the men being marched down to the bathing ground in squads, and allowed to remain only a few minutes (from 5 to 10) in the water. This length of time is sufficient for all purposes of ablution. *But no bathing should on any account be permitted immediately after meals, nor at evening.* The habit is a dangerous one in many ways, and should be discountenanced.

By the various hygienic measures above enumerated, when systematized and carried into effect, a corps of young recruits may be so strengthened and hardened as to enable them, after a month's sojourn in barracks, to take the field with very fair chances;

whereas, without such gradual breaking in, the new volunteer, passing suddenly from the counting-room to the ranks of an army, is likely to wilt under the first day's march; to be sickened by the meagreness of his new diet, and to be found in the hospital rather than on the battle-field when the enemy makes his appearance.

CHAPTER IV.

HYGIENE OF BARRACKS.

Barracks, not being castles of defence but simply habitations, should always be constructed with particular reference to hygienic requirements. But, in order to be habitations of comfort, they must first be habitations of health. No false economy should be permitted to interfere with this most important of all considerations. And it should be remembered also that it is easier to provide for it during the construction of an edifice than by remodelling it afterwards.

The paramount necessities of all buildings destined for dwellings, are a free and constant supply of pure air, and a due exposure to sunlight.* Both these necessities are increased by the number of hu-

* As an illustration of the importance of sunlight, it is stated that, in the citadel of Ghent, in 1845 and 1846, those companies which lodged in subterranean apartments had twice as many sick as those which lodged above ground. Few persons outside of the medical profession really appreciate the deteriorating influences produced upon the human constitution by depriving it of the vivifying stimulus of sunlight. The very air becomes in some measure deteriorated by its long absence.

man beings inhabiting them; but the former, at least, is indispensable from the very start. Insufficiency of air and its consequent depravation is not, however, one of those active causes which kill on the spot. But it is the more dangerous, because of the insidious effects produced upon the constitution, and the inability to detect them ere serious mischief is done. The general alterations in the system produced by it manifest themselves in the form of chronic glandular degenerations, like scrofula, phthisis, &c., or of such contagious maladies as typhus, variola, purulent ophthalmia, and dysentery. Statistics have long shown the large proportion of deaths from phthisis and typhus obtaining in all armies, and if this be so, then what better cause can be assigned for it, than that of overcrowding and ill ventilation in barracks, huts, and tents?

Dry, airy sites, with a proper slope for drainage, and an exposure to sunlight, are the best ones for barracks. They should not, when erected in cities, be placed in densely populated portions, or be surrounded by high buildings.

Whatever the size of the building or material of construction, the walls should be thick, in order to insure perfect dryness, and windows of sufficient size (the larger the better) should abound on all sides. It is better to have the building with as long a front as possible. If wings are necessary they may be added, but never so as to form a perfect square with an inclosed court-yard, as this latter is in such cases always a nursery of dampness.

3

All mess-rooms, guard-rooms, and dormitories should have an altitude of at least 15 feet, be thoroughly ventilated, and be situated so as to receive the sunshine during some portion of the day. The walls and ceilings should be plastered and painted, so as to exclude dampness and admit of cleansing.

The best size for dormitories, consistent with health, is such as will contain from 12 to 14 beds. But the number of occupants in any room should always be so calculated as to afford to each man 400 cubic feet of air, with ventilation adequate to supplying him with 40 cubic feet of fresh air per hour.* For this purpose, windows must be partially opened at night, and fully during the day, whenever the weather permits.

The bedstead should be of iron, and single, and the bed should consist of a thick straw pallet and pillow. Sheets are cleanly and should not be dispensed with in barracks. All beds should be turned, and bedding aired daily. But when soldiers are preparing

* In illustration of the dangers which ever attend *overcrowding*, in even the best-regulated barracks, may be cited the facts observed in the military hospital of Versailles, from 1843 to 1847, where an annual epidemic of typhoid fever was seen to prevail among patients brought from the garrison of St. Cloud. This epidemic declared itself annually a few days after the arrival of the king at the palace of St. Cloud, and disappeared immediately on his departure. Ordinarily the garrison there consisted of from 400 to 500 men, but the king's advent increased it to 1,200! The troops were consequently overcrowded in all their quarters, and typhoid fever invariably manifested itself. This fact is a significant commentary upon the deleterious influences that always attend upon overcrowded establishments, and will apply to gaols, workhouses, and pauper asylums, as well as to barracks.

for immediate service in the field, they should be gradually weaned from the use of sheets, and even the straw pallet, and made to rough it on the floor in their blankets, with knapsacks for pillows.

All *wash-rooms*, *mess-rooms*, and *guard-rooms* should be on the ground floor, and the former should be tiled, with a sloping floor, and a drain running through the centre. Around the wash-sinks, wooden gratings should be placed for the men to stand on while performing their ablutions.

All *privies*, *urinals*, and *cess-pools* should be daily disinfected in the absence of any stream of water running through them.* They should communicate with a subterranean sewer, and be under semi-weekly observation by the medical officer of the post.

There should be an ante-chamber to the guard-room, with a fire kept burning in it during wet weather, where men coming in from out-door duties may put off and dry their *wet* outside garments.

The barrack-yard should be planted with trees as much as practicable. *Evergreens* (pines in particular) are preferable on the score of health, as well as room.

No copper or lead vessels should be used in cooking, except when *tinned*, and their condition should be frequently inspected by the medical officer of the post.

All floors, except those of bed-rooms, should be

* Among the cheap disinfectants may be mentioned the Chloride and Sulphate of Lime (Gypsum), *in powder*, and Sulphate of Iron (Green Copperas), *in solution*, and Sulphuric and Muriatic Acid Gas.

daily scrubbed in fine weather, as well as swept. The sweeping must never be omitted; the scrubbing may be, in wet weather. Floors should be kept painted. Ceilings and walls should be whitewashed as often as once a month.

The men should not be allowed to wear their shoes to their dormitories, but should leave them in their lockers when they go to bed.

A urinal should be fixed near the door of each dormitory, and used only at night.

CHAPTER V.

THE MARCH.

A MILITARY march is one of the most fatiguing of all exercises in walking, and in its effects upon the system must not be judged of by any similar exertion singly undertaken in civil life. It is one thing to walk alone, and as you please, with as little or as much load as you may prefer, with the privilege of resting as often and as long as you please, and of going only as far as inclination prompts; and it is quite another and a different thing to march in ranks, and always in the same place, keeping step with one before you, treading amid clouds of dust, clad warmly, and heavily burthened with accoutrements, unable to stop at the first promptings of fatigue, and compelled to accomplish a certain per diem of locomotion. Such is a military march. Thus the weak must keep up with the strong, the man of short stride with the one of long; and the very regularity of the step does, when prolonged, tend to make it wearisome and exhausting.

Another consideration when marching also deserves to be thought of, and that is the privilege of swinging the arm, which, as a balance to that side of the body opposite the musket, becomes an imperious necessity for comfort. Although forbidden on occasions like *drills* and *parades* as being ungraceful, the restriction should, in kindness to the soldier, be removed on the march. Wherever it is practicable the men should be allowed to march freely, and without the restraint of well-dressed ranks. In this way the march is relieved of much of its harassing character, and becomes a salutary and tonifying exercise. The men are more cheerful, more ambitious, and capable of a higher measure of endurance. The skill of a commander cannot be better shown than in preserving the spirits of his troops while causing them to perform long marches.

One of the pre-requisite conditions to all good marching is the possession of a pair of good feet. The feet in fact are the battle-charger of the infantry-soldier, and serve to carry him through the march and the fray. It becomes important, therefore, that he should keep them in good order. For this purpose, the pattern of all army shoes should present us with a *broad sole* as the first preventive to cramping the feet; a *stout single-soled* shoe made of light kip leather, laced around the ankle, combines all the elements of lightness and durability, protection to the foot, and support to the ankle, which can be desired in any shoe. Over such an article, a gaiter would not be needed, although, if possible, they should be worn, and when so, the shoe would not need to reach so high.

In the *disposition* of a march certain *hygienic* as well as strategic elements enter. For it is evident that if the character of the march be so imprudently designed as (by *excess of length, exposure to storms, roughness of country, and omissions of intervals of rest and refreshment*) to fatigue and harass troops, a commander will succeed only in breaking down his soldiers, so that the more he marches, and the nearer he approaches the enemy, the less fit he will be to encounter him. In an enemy's country it is always better to make *short* marches, and to keep troops fresh, than to attempt long ones, which only result in swelling the sick list. Fatigue and exhaustion are as destructive to courage, as they are to endurance, and when General *Debility* takes command of an army, the possession of rifled-cannon and Minié balls are of little avail to it. Tonicity of muscular fibre is like dryness to powder; the more there is of it, the greater the destructive power engendered, while flaccidity on the one hand and dampness on the other, render both these ministers of war absolutely inert.

Too long, too rapid, or ill-regulated marches, are ever apt to occasion sickness, and to provoke those inevitable results of over-fatigue, complete prostration, and internal congestions. The fact is so often made manifest in the increase of the hospital list, which ever follows upon ill-regulated and fatiguing marches, that it hardly needs repetition. We find in the *Archives de Medecine Militaire** the following

* Tome 9, page 15.

incident most strongly illustrative of the point under review. Two brigades arrived at the same dépôt; the one had made protracted marches, partly by night; the other short and slow ones, always by day, and here was the result as furnished by the hospital-record:

Marching by Long Stages Partly by Night.

2d Regiment had	60	days of	sickness.
4th " "	41	"	"
6th (1st batt'n)	43	"	"

Marching by Short Stages Always by Day.

1st Regiment had	32	days of	sickness.
6th (2d & 3d bat.)	14	"	"
12th Reg't had	19	"	"
3d Chass.(foot) "	23	"	"

Thus those who made long marches, and partly by night, lost *twice* as much time by sickness as those who made short marches and always by day, a significant commentary upon the hygiene of exercise.

The hygienic considerations that should regulate a march are those of *season*, *weather*, *physical character of country*, *and condition* of troops. The same length of daily march which might be accomplished in winter, could not with safety be gone over in summer; nor in a rain-storm as on a dry day; nor in a flat, sandy country, as among hills; nor with young and raw troops as with veterans. The great object being not simply to transport men a certain distance, so much as to present them upon a certain spot in *fighting order*, officers will see the propriety of never willingly undertaking *forced* marches, as the risks of breaking down new troops are too great to be lightly incurred. Particularly is this the case in hot weather, when all the disadvantages in dress and weight, under which the soldier labors, render him doubly accessible to fatigue and disease.* In him the excess of heat at the surface generated by prolonged exercise, finds no ready means of escape through his thick clothing. The weight of the knapsack, and the constriction of the chest caused by its cross-belt, greatly impede the function of respiration, and give rise to acute disorders of its organs. Pneumonia, pleurisy, bronchitis, &c., attest the ill effects that flow from these causes.

When marching under the conditions of a high temperature, the soldier should be allowed to *unbutton his coat*, and to turn down his collar, the distances between the ranks should be widened† to twice or even

* Asphyxia supervening upon extreme fatigue, has been frequently noticed in the French army in Africa, particularly during the prevalence of the sirocco. Even *mania* has followed upon protracted marching; and in General Bugeaud's expedition in 1836, *eleven suicides* were recorded.

† All who have ever been in a crowd on a hot day, know how suffocating is the atmosphere created by a body of men close together, and radiating about them the corporeal emanations which always accompany even insensible perspiration. But when clothing becomes saturated under such circumstances with visible perspiration, we have here a real human miasma developed, under the combined influences of heat, moisture, and volatilized animal

thrice the usual measure, and he should be relieved of all superfluous baggage; or if that cannot be done, the distances marched should be short,* and gone over early in the day.

The *slow pace* (3 miles the hour) is the proper one for all ordinary occasions, as infantry can then keep up with cavalry: besides which the march is easier for all, and there are fewer laggards. At the expiration of the first hour a halt of *ten* minutes will be found of service.

At the expiration of the second hour a halt of fifteen minutes should be allowed, and the men be permitted to lie down if they choose, unsling knapsacks, unbutton coats, but not to remove them, and take off their shoes. Neither should they be allowed to drink immoderately of cold water from any stream hard by. The canteens should be filled before starting, and suffice until the final halt of the day; and in order to keep their contents cool, they should be covered with a piece of white cotton cloth kept constantly wet. By dipping the canteen in any water during the halt, and allowing a few minutes evaporation from the cloth to occur, the contained water will be found much lowered in temperature. Another halt of ten minutes at

matter. *Thirteen* inches, the space allowed between the ranks, is not sufficient in hot weather, and on a march. Men should never be so near as to *smell* each other.

* All authorities are agreed that when long journeys are to be accomplished, the daily marches should be short. A long one at the beginning has been known to essentially defeat the object of the journey, by breaking down a large number of men, and unfitting them for active duty.

the expiration of the third hour should take place as before. With the fourth hour of march, exclusive of stops, the column will have accomplished from 12 to 15 miles according to the step taken. Twelve miles is considered an ordinary day's march in the British army, and fifteen in the French.* Considering the American constitution as being more nearly allied to the British than to the French, we should say that 12 miles per diem was the extent to which any large column should be pushed during the summer months.

Should the exigencies of the service require that a longer march be accomplished, some additional precautionary measures will be necessary. After having marched the usual time of four hours, the column should be halted for a full hour, the men be made to take off stockings, to roll up pantaloons, and to wash their faces, necks, feet, and legs. After which a ration of biscuit and coffee should be served out. By these simple and ever accessible means the men will be sufficiently refreshed to march an hour or two longer without much risk to health.

When making a halt, the officer in command should avoid deep, sandy cuts, or places where there is not a free circulation of air. Open ground, somewhat sheltered by trees, and near running water, is the better place; but as all these qualities are not

* When it is remembered that the soldier on reaching his camping ground cannot at once rest himself, but must prepare his lodgment, procure wood and water, and do an infinity of small duties, not to speak of guard-mounting, it will be seen that 12 miles a day is a sufficient march at any ordinary time.

easily found, the officer will have to exercise his own judgment in all cases relating to choice of localities.

Young troops should, in marching, be placed in the van of the main body. It will be found that they do not experience so much fatigue in leading, as in following the column; and in case of a skirmish, they behave better, and are more self-reliant, from the consciousness of having older troops in their rear to support them. The moral effect thus produced upon young soldiers exerts a direct and dynamic influence upon their physical courage; stimulates them to renewed efforts, enables them to endure fatigue much better, and makes them strive to win the respect of their older brethren in arms, by sharing in common all their labors.

Season and Weather.—The rule of marching with reference to season and weather, should be this, viz.: that in summer the day's march should be accomplished before noon. The same rule holds good when marches *must* be made in wet weather, as that enables troops to collect wood for fires during the afternoon; to provide shelter for the night, and to dry themselves before lying down. As a general thing, however, troops should not be marched, unless the urgency demands it, in wet weather. The dampness of so much clothing, much of it already saturated with organic emanations, the heat of so many bodies marching and perspiring in immediate contact, and the subsequent crowding of half-a-dozen wet, reeking men into one tent with every aperture closed, present all the necessary conditions for the development of epidemic disease. We must not be surprised under such circumstances, and when the march is continued for many days, to meet with dysentery and typhoid fever. They are the legitimate offspring of such morbific influences.

Character of Country.—It is easier to make long marches in a hilly than in a level, sandy country. The reason is obvious. The muscles used in walking are not rested simply by inaction, but also by variety of action; and that variety is best obtained by changes in the configuration of the ground over which we march. Besides which, the mind is more stimulated by the variety of scenery afforded it in a hilly country. There is no "weary waste expanding to the skies," around it, to fatigue the eye, and weary the senses with a dull, monotonous sameness. But, on the contrary, every hill-top presents a new vista, and stimulates to fresh exertion. This stimulation, born of a pure, highly oxygenated air, gives elasticity to the spirits, causes the flagging energies to revive, and sends a thrill of ardor through the soldier's heart. It was thus that the view of the plains of Italy from the summits of the Alps fired the hearts of Napoleon's soldiers, and made them forget the fatigues of their hard climbing.

Condition of Troops.—In order to accomplish a successful march, troops should be "fresh" at the start. A great battle, or the execution of laborious field-works, should not be immediately followed by a march of those who have taken active parts in these operations. A day's intervening rest and refreshment will do much towards recruiting the energies of soldiers who have thus exhausted themselves. For although it may at times be necessary to "push on" immediately after a battle, yet it will generally be found that this can only be done with impunity by victorious troops, buoyed up by the stimulus of high spirits. But that great risk of overtasking men is always run in such cases, none will pretend to deny; and while it may be justifiable in the defeated to escape at any and every hazard to health, the same cannot be pleaded by the victorious.

Troops should never be marched *fasting*. A ration of *coffee* and *biscuit*, if time admits of nothing else, should always be served to the men before *starting* in the morning. This is particularly necessary in malarious districts, and should never be omitted. The French will often make a morning march on nothing but bread and coffee. Our troops require more; but without this much at least, they should not be made to march.

Convalescents should be spared as much as possible on the march. Walking is fatiguing enough for them. Their knapsacks and arms should be placed with the baggage, and they near it. In crossing rivers, every precaution should be employed against their being wetted, as this exposure, added to fatigue, would speedily return them to the hospital. Refreshments should also be administered to them during the march, in order to preserve their strength; and at each halt they should, if possible, be allowed to lie down in the baggage-wagons. Extra covering should be furnished them at night, and they should never sleep without a tent. With these precautions they will be able to follow the march, and even be strengthened by it, so as shortly to resume their places in the ranks. There is not so much danger of malingering among volunteers enlisted for a few months, as among regulars enlisted for several years. Among the former, the desire is rather to push on, than to lag behind. While in the latter, military ardor is apt to become somewhat abated by the feeling that several years of service as professional soldiers still lies before them.

CHAPTER VI.

THE CAMP.

It is unnecessary in a hygienic point of view to speak of all the varieties of camps upon which military authorities dwell. These classifications being purely strategic, have no special application to our subject. We will limit ourselves, therefore, to the two simple divisions of *flying* and *intrenched* camps.

In the Flying Camp, which, as its name implies, is to be occupied only for a short period, and where no tents are to be erected, care should be taken to select a spot combining as many of the qualities of *dryness* of soil, proximity to *fresh water,* and *shelter from winds,* as possible. These are the three hygienic elements which should govern officers in the selection of its site. But the short time during which the camp is to be occupied, will not require that the same stringency in hygienic precautions should be enforced as in a permanent camp. Its temporary character relieves it from many of those dangers of epidemic visitation which hover over intrenched camps. Still, from the greater exposure to the weather in it, sporadic cases of disease will soon appear, if no preventive measures are employed. It is the part of wisdom, then, to provide against these, by hedging the troops about with as many safeguards to health as the nature of their circumstances admits of.

In selecting the site of an encampment, all proximity to *swamps* should be avoided, unless some intervening rising ground, or a dense belt of woods exists, to arrest the current of miasma which constantly flows from them. Experience seems to show that exposed heights, five and six hundred feet to leeward of swamps, are more susceptible to the influences of their miasma than a level or undulating plain half that distance off.* Whenever, therefore, it becomes necessary to occupy such places, fires should be kindled on the windward side, or the men should be made to wear overcoats when mounting guard at night. They should not be exercised fasting, and a more stimulating diet must be given them.

Dryness of Soil.—This is not simply essential, but also indispensable, to the health of troops. Men cannot sleep nor even lie with impunity upon damp ground. Their beds, whether it be earth or board, must be dry, so must their blankets. Double safety would undoubtedly be secured by an india-rubber blanket, which neither gets wet, nor allows the dampness of the earth to penetrate it. Hemlock or pine boughs make good enough beds; but even if no contact of the person with the damp earth occurs, the

* Dr. Jackson "On Armies."

emanations from such a soil, particularly in hot weather, cannot be otherwise than deleterious.

Wherever it is permissible, *fires should be lighted* and kept burning all night on the windward side of the camp. They serve, in some degree, to purify the air, (*Est in ipsis ignibus medica vis.*—Pliny,) but, more than all, to temper it. In musquito-breeding or malarious regions, they will be found particularly serviceable.

SHELTER FROM WINDS.—This is an important consideration in the selection of a spot for a flying camp, especially when the troops have been exposed to the wet during the day, or the weather be cold. Winds passing over damp clothing, rapidly lower the temperature of the surface of the body, and dispose to inflammatory disorders. It is important to guard against this source of danger by a natural shelter, as well as by fires.

In the INTRENCHED CAMP, which is designed to be a more permanent habitation for troops, other and stricter rules of hygiene must be enforced. In the selection of its site, and wherever practicable, the same considerations as to dryness of soil and proximity to fresh water should obtain. Providing the soil be not argillaceous, the presence of some moisture (springiness) is no cause for apprehension; but the locality of the camp should always be such as to admit of complete surface drainage either by direct flowage or by percolation. The result of all observation shows that a light, sandy soil, bordering on the banks of a wooded stream, affords the healthiest of all camping-grounds; and in selecting such a site, the medical staff should always be consulted.

The first hygienic requirement in a camp, as in a city, is that its population shall not be overcrowded in its various lodging-places. To prevent this, wherever tents are used, they should be capacious enough to afford each occupant, at the very least, 108 cubic ($6 \times 6 \times 3$) feet of air, with a renewal of 40 cubic feet per hour. The English "Bell" tent with a diameter of 13 ft. 8, and an altitude of *ten* feet, affords to each one of its occupants 146 cubic feet. The Portsmouth hut, which is much larger, and affords room for 25 men, gives to each the same amount (146 feet) of breathing space. Yet large as this seems to be, there is good reason to believe that it is still insufficient in stormy weather, when necessity requires an almost entire closing of the tent. To obviate the risks to health from this practice, they should be made with only partial sides (drops) to be used in slantwise rains, or fewer men should be assigned to their occupancy. Without some such precautions, tents are apt to become foul to a degree scarcely credible, and in this way to afford nurseries for the generation of epidemic diseases. Authorities differ greatly in their various estimates of the value of tents as hygienic auxiliaries; and certainly, without a more rigid sanitary surveillance than has heretofore been enforced in camps, the evils directly traceable to them have not been unduly magnified. But the same might, with equal justice, be said of tenant-houses; and yet the poor must be *housed*, even at the expense of health. We imagine the fault does not so much lie in the tent itself as in the mode in which it is occupied, and the want of due ventilation and the negligence in cleanliness among its occupants. When these two objections are removed, we can find nothing in the structure itself to condemn.

Still, it is an undoubted fact that the contact of many warm bodies with the humid earth, as in a tent, by first raising the temperature of the contained atmosphere, and causing an ascent of moisture saturated with organic emanations, produces the best conditions for the development of disease. And those diseases, by the very asthenic and typhoid types which they assume, clearly enough indicate the sources of their origin. The camp dysenteries of the Crimea were most generally of this type, even as all fevers become modified by the medium in which they have been developed, independent of any ingenerate character of their own. The daily observation of such facts as these, multiplied and reduplicated in the hospital records of all armies in modern times, should make us blush with indignation at that stupid apathy which has so long permitted *preventible* disease to decimate the flower of every army.

The late Dr. Jackson, surgeon-general to the British army, was of opinion that tents were not essential to health; and certainly as formerly managed, they were among its greatest enemies. He gave the preference to *huts*, alleging their superiority on the point of cleanliness and ventilation, and even asserted that men could do well without either. We are not prepared to say as much as that, believing as we do in the superiority of a well-ordered tent over all other kinds of shelter. But for safety's sake it should only have *partial* sides, not close walls, a trench dug completely around it to receive and lead away the rain; and not less than *four* feet should intervene between the stakes of each tent.

Every occupied tent, at night, should have a large portion of its doorway, or during a storm some other aperture on the leeward side, open, for purposes of ventilation. The corporals of each guard in making their rounds should see to the enforcement of this rule, also that the men do not smoke in the tent. It would also be well, were it possible, to insist upon the men's blankets being inspected at night to see that they are not *wet* when used as coverings. And when the guard is relieved in rainy weather, and before a soldier retires to his quarters he should, if he has used his blanket, be given a dry one in exchange, in which to sleep.

The floor of each tent should be covered with an india-rubber, or painted canvas cloth, which should form part of the camp-equipage just as much as the tent itself. In this day of meridional civilization, it is unjustifiable to omit any thing which can protect troops from the risk of sleeping on damp, cold ground. Tents must have floors; wood is cheap, but bulky to transport, and, besides, becomes saturated with organic emanations. India-rubber, on the contrary, is cheap, light, and always clean.

To each twenty men there should be allowed a

night-bucket with a cover, to serve as a *urinal, and to be used only at night.* This is cleanlier than to allow men to ease themselves on the ground in the vicinity of the tents, (as the soil soon becomes foul and offensive,) while, at the same time, it relieves them from the necessity of going to the privies at the extreme rear of the regiment in wet and stormy weather.

The regimental privies or sinks should be encircled by bushes, and every evening a portion of the earth dug out of them should be thrown in. A *special privy should be allotted to the dejections coming from hospital patients;* and this should, when much sickness prevails, be daily disinfected.

Every tent should be thoroughly aired daily; and all straw, hay, or other bedding contained in it should, on every fair day, be taken out, and aired in the sun. But whenever the same becomes mouldy or offensive by age, it must be thrown away. The blankets of the men should also be daily aired and sunned.

Once a week they should be made to wash themselves and change their body clothing, and an opportunity be also given them to wash their soiled clothes. Regular wash-days, for this purpose, when practicable should be appointed, in order to avoid the accumulation of soiled clothing in the tents.

At least twice in every week, the surgeon or his assistant should make a sanitary inspection of all the tents, kitchens, and sinks throughout the camp. Each company should detail two corporals to attend him in the inspection of its own tents. Neither the day nor the hour of the inspection should be announced beforehand.

The medical officer, at the same time, should inspect all provisions in actual use ; the barrels, boxes, pots, or cans in which they are kept; and the power should be given him to order any thing to be destroyed with whose sanitary condition he is dissatisfied.

Guard-Mounting.—As sleep is among the most indispensable of our necessities, so its loss is followed by a degree of lassitude and discomfort amounting in many to actual suffering. Although all do not immediately experience the same ill effects from its loss, yet practically the effect is in the end the same, whenever the absence of sleep is protracted. The young and the weakly succumb first, the mature and the healthy follow them also at no inconsiderable interval of time. Superadded to the fatigues of the day, the duty of mounting guard is, among young troops, the severest task which can be imposed upon them. Nothing, in fact, will sooner destroy the health of youth than privation of a due amount of sleep; and it is on this account that it becomes important to allot the duty of guard-mounting to those who can stand it best.

As a hygienic rule founded in a strict economy of strength, the youngest troops (from 18 to 21) should not be put on guard at night after a march, or battle, although they may, when a regiment is permanently encamped. But in any event, the first hours of the night should not be assigned to them. The mature of age are more wakeful during the early part of night, while the young are more disposed to sleep. Hence the young should be put on duty during the last watches of the night, and when they have already received all needed benefit from sleep. The older men will, in like manner, receive their measure of rest at the time when nature most prompts them to seek it, so that by thus following the dictates of natural appetites the health of all classes may be preserved.

Sleep is, indeed, such an imperative necessity with the young, that to rob them of it is to strike the most cruel blow at their physical vigor. The loss of a meal, or a long march, will not produce such depressing effects upon their health as the loss of one night's sleep. And the nervous energy being thus lowered in tone, the system becomes readily accessible to the seeds of any endemic or epidemic malady. It is rendered more sensitive to the impressions of cold, to the influence of malaria, and, in fact, to all extraneous circumstances. Timely circumspection on the part of officers is needed here, to prevent injuring troops, which, surrounded by all other hygienic conditions, may yet, through a negligent disregard of the proper allotment of sleep necessary to meet the requirements of different ages, be debilitated and unfitted for the successful performance of their duties in the field.

CHAPTER VII.

THE FOOD.

The diet of the soldier plays an important part in the economy of his military life. For, in contradistinction to the civilian, it is not sufficient that his food should simply sustain life, but it should also be possessed of such qualities as to develop in him a high degree of animal spirits. It should give vigor to his health through appropriate stimulating virtues, and leave behind a measure of positive strength due to its inherent tonic properties. All have observed the diversities which national character assumes under varieties of diet. The difference between the *meat* and *wheat*-fed European, and the *rice*-fed Hindoo; the *maize*-fed Mexican, and the *fish* and *yam*-fed South Sea Islander, in all the qualities of intellectuality, strength of body, and persevering energy and endurance, is too marked to have escaped notice. It may be stated as a universal rule, that the conquering races of the earth have always been the best fed races, not indeed in the sense of luxurious indulgence, but in the possession and use of those aliments which impress upon the system a vigorous tone, and thus develop physical courage. The same rule also obtains among animals. The high bred hunter, the racehorse, or the roadster, all attest through the manner in which they do their appointed work, the tonifying quality of their diet.

All these truisms point directly to the necessity of making the soldier's dietary an important part of the discipline of an army, as well as of its hygiene. In an economic point of view, it may be said that a weak soldier is no soldier, costing the state more to support him than his services are worth. True wisdom, and true economy, therefore, lies in furnishing him with such qualities of aliment as will keep his physical energies always at par. His life is peculiarly exposed to incessant causes of debility and to attacks of disease. He is suddenly translated from civic life, with its regular, generally controllable duties, to a military life with its fatiguing drills, marches, guard-mountings, irregularities in times of occupation and eating, overcrowding in tents and barracks, exposure to heat and moisture, and vicissitudes of climate, all of which none will certainly pretend to say are calculated to strengthen, so much as they are to shock, and to enfeeble the system. Such an individual of all others, needs a tonic and recuperating diet, and unless he finds it, very soon takes his place in a hospital ward with broken health. It is far cheaper to feed him well in the field than to nurse him in the hospital.

In order, therefore, to be serviceable to the state,

soldiers must be fed well. In order to enable them to bear the fatigues of marching, to breast the vicissitudes of weather, and to encounter, unaffected, the changes of climate, their bodies must be nourished with particular reference to developing a high muscular tone. Experience has shown that a *mixed diet*, in which animal food preponderates, is that most conducive to this result. Consequently it is to such a form of diet that we must look for maintaining the health and utility of an army. Nothing is more true than that good food is as much a munition of war as good powder.

On examining the bill of rations of our army, two important facts strike us at the outset. The first is the narrow range of the dietary, amounting in its monotonous uniformity almost to *exclusivism*, and second its too often *unseasonable* character. Now, in these days of easy transportation, there is clearly no justification on the plea of economy for either, while science and experience conspire to condemn both as the fruitful sources of mischief to health. There is an instinctive craving for variety of food in all organisms, and however good any single article may in itself be, its continued and exclusive use for any length of time is sure to inspire disgust, and consequently to impair its nutritive character. In such cases men may be filled with it, and yet not fed by it, because nutrition depends upon assimilation, and assimilation upon that tone of the digestive canal which manifests itself through taste and *relish*. What we cease to relish we are neither apt to assimilate, nor to be nourished by. The very craving for variety in food is thus made an index of the necessity of a change in its character to our organism.

Again, we may have, relatively speaking, a strong diet at any period of the year, but in order also to be a healthy one, it must conform itself in a measure to the requirements of the season. Hence, in an army, every thing, whether labor, food, or clothing, should be regulated first of all by the necessities of the season. And inasmuch as most campaigns, or active operations in the field, take place in summer, and may, besides, extend into hot climates, the soldier's dietary should be so arranged as to enable him not only to meet the exigencies of his own laborious calling, but also to resist the constitutional influences of a debilitating season. The object should be to have each article nutritious, without at the same time inducing any predisposition to diseases of the season. In a word, the dietary should be both alimentary and corrective.

A diet consisting simply of flesh and cereals, although eminently nourishing, could not be endured throughout the summer with impunity. And if that flesh were salted, it would greatly increase the tendency to disease. The proximate principles of organic matter must always be present, but they should change their proportions and relative position in the scale of our rations to meet climatic variations. As now established, the soldier's fare is a true winter diet, and rich in elements well suited to meet the requirements of respiration, under a low temperature.

In summer, on the contrary, the excess of carbon furnished by it to the lungs beyond what they can dispose of, imposes additional duties of elimination upon the liver, and tends unduly to excite this organ. A predisposition to biliary disorders is consequently engendered.

In order to counteract the ill effects of so alkalescent a diet in summer, recourse must be had to fruits and vegetable acids. These, with spices, are nature's own correctives. Both, also admitting of preservation, should be regularly included among army supplies. By a proper disposition of his diet, man lives as healthfully under the equator as under the pole. The East Indian with his rice and yams, and the Esquimaux with his seal-blubber and putrid fish, are both healthy enough in their respective climates, but let them once change residences without changing their diet, and what would be the consequence? The Esquimaux would be attacked with putrid fever, and the West Indian would die of inanition.

We perceive from this the absolute necessity of modifying all forms of diet in such a way as to accommodate them to the physiological requirements of varying seasons. For habit is not acquirable as against the laws of chemical combination, and no man can become habituated to doing that with impunity, which, being a violation of the physiological laws of his system, is, by its frequent admonitions of pain, notifying him of the evil about to overtake him.

As the ration bill now stands, it presents us with too concentrated a form of diet for continued use. It abounds in *fibrine*, *gluten*, and *fat*, without, however, a sufficiency in *starch*, *mucilage*, *gelatin*, and *acids*. *Aromatic herbs* and *spices*, without which health cannot for any length of time be preserved, particularly in hot climates or seasons, are entirely omitted, while *fat pork*, an article contra-indicated in summer both by the state of the appetite and the physiological necessities of the system, stands as the sheet anchor of its animal food. Lean hams, shoulders and sides, or jerked beef, should be substituted in its stead. In the arrangement of the summer dietary, it should be remembered that animal *fats* must take a subordinate rank, and *starchy* food, *esculent* roots, *aromatics*, and *vegetable* acids be allowed to preponderate.

It is not from the *quantity* of food digested, so much as by the power of assimilating it, that mankind are nourished. A pound and a half of pork or beef per day would sicken and debilitate the Arab whose handful of dates enables him, between sun and sun, to perform fatiguing exercises; while the same amount of flesh would hardly suffice to keep alive an Esquimaux bantling. The reason for this difference rests solely in the function of assimilation, a function which is of all others the most speedily affected and deranged by too exclusive and concentrated a diet. The story of the peasant who broke his thigh, and while in the hospital fell into a complete *marasmus* when fed on beef-tea, custards, rice-milk and wine, and only recovered when restored to his original diet of black bread, greens, fish, and oil, is a pointed illustration of the *innutritious effects* of too *nutritious* a dietary long persisted in.

Now, because soldiers have hard work to do, we must not imagine that all they require in food is simply what chemists have ascertained to be *nutritive* reparative qualities. They cannot be fed like steam-engines, by just so many pounds of this or that kind of fuel daily and unvaryingly administered. A man losing 2 or 3 pounds in weight by perspiration to-day, could not be restored to-night by simply gorging him with a like weight of beef, pork, or bread. In the presence of vital forces, the conduct of organic functions cannot be regulated by chemical formulæ born of the laboratory. No narrow methodism is tolerable here. We must follow experience alone; and experience everywhere shows that in the healthy health is alone to be preserved by a *liberal, mixed diet.* If we would preserve the health of our troops we must amplify the range of their dietary. It may cost a little more, and but a little more, yet that little is an hundred per cent. less than the cost of nursing a sick man, paying him wages besides, and over all, losing the benefit of his presence on the battle-field. We fancy that no economist would be long in determining which measure of the two is cheapest in the end.

Experience having demonstrated that no single substance, be it animal or vegetable, when exclusively indulged in for any length of timé, can support the human body in health, but that the continuous use of the same food produces debility of the digestive apparatus, satiety, and consequent faulty nutrition, it becomes indispensable to the health of soldiers that each meal should be composed of a due admixture of *animal* and *vegetable* substances, and further that the dietary should be so arranged as to avoid repetition and *sameness* in the articles daily used.

It is also established that, in order to maintain healthy digestion, all alimentary substances should occasionally be accompanied by condiments of a *saline, spicy,* or *aromatic* and *acid* character. Salt, pepper, and the aromatic principles of certain vegetables like onions, parsley, thyme, and garlick; the spices proper, cloves, ginger, &c., or the vegetable acids, sorrel, vinegar, &c., when taken in concert with our food, tend to promote its more perfect elaboration, or to correct a disposition to fermentation and putrescency.

In a country blessed with plenty like our own, with means of transportation at every door, and where almost every village sends its company of volunteers, it is not difficult to provide a dietary like that which follows. The articles superadded to the regular army rations could be easily made up for each company *in its own home*, and forwarded to its quarters in the field. Thus barrels of apples, potatoes, onions and carrots, where troops are at a depot, might easily be sent them. It is understood that the Government makes no objection to their transmission, and nothing but willingness is therefore wanted on the part of patriotic committees at home.

In alimentary rank animal food must take precedence of all other kinds. Next to this come bread and farinaceous articles, and lastly esculent roots and spices. The order of their disposition in any dietary should be nearly as follows:

FOR A WINTER DIET.	FOR A SUMMER DIET.
Pork, 3 days in a week.	Beef, 3 days.
Beef,* 3 days in a week.	Mutton, 3 days.
Mutton, or Salt Fish, 1 day in a week.	Pork, or Salt Fish, 1 day.
Flour,† Wheat and Indian.	Flour.
Beans, 2 days in a week.	Beans or Barley, 1 day.
Potatoes, 2 days in a week.	Rice, 3 days.
Esculent Roots, Pickled Cabbage, and dried Fruits, 3 times a week.	Dried or fresh Fruits, or Pickled Cabbage, 3 days.
Coffee, twice daily.	Coffee, twice daily.
Sugar—Spices.	Sugar—Spices.

With regard to *quality*, it may be said that *fresh* meats are always more nourishing than salt, dried, or

* The cheapness of beef in our country renders it unnecessary that I should say aught on the subject of *horse-flesh*, now so much in vogue in some parts of Europe. It is unquestionably proved to be highly palatable, nutritious, and in nowise inferior to beef as an article of alimentation. Philosophers have fed upon it, and detailed with rapture its good qualities, and one of them, Geoffroy de St. Hilaire, has consecrated its merits in a volume of considerable size.

† It is more economical, as well as healthy, to feed soldiers on *stale*, rather than on fresh bread. Less of the former is apt to be eaten, and less suffices to nourish them. By stale is to be understood bread which has been out of the oven, and exposed to the air *at least* 24 hours.

It would be better also if the bread could be made of *wheat-middlings*, instead of fine flour, as a large percentage of nutritive matter (gluten) is removed with the husk in the process of bolting. Indian meal should also be occasionally mixed with fine flour in smoked, which latter are also more indigestible. That the flesh of grown animals exceeds in nutritive value that of the young, and that moderately fat meats are the best of all.

With regard to vegetables and fruits the same rules apply, to a certain extent. Fresh vegetables are always preferable to dry or preserved ones. Farinaceous vegetables like potatoes, beans, and peas, are more nourishing than roots and grasses, such as cabbage, spinage, &c. Nevertheless, the system occasionally requires such articles as cabbages, turnips, onions, carrots, &c., and their peculiarly *corrective* qualities are called for to mitigate the scorbutic tendencies of too exclusive a diet of salt meat.* The acid fruits, like dried apples and peaches, when fresh ones cannot be obtained, should find a regular place in the

making bread. The popular aversion to dark-colored bread, founded on the supposition of its lesser amount of nourishment, is a gross error. The best soldiers in the world are fed on dark-colored bread.

The importance of *good bread* to health is so universally recognized that I have deemed it unnecessary to say aught upon the subject. There are frequent enough complaints about the quality of the beef issued to troops, but I imagine that there is full as much dereliction in the matter of bread. Now, certainly, there can be no excuse for either, although, of the two, I entertain no doubt that bad bread works more silent mischief than bad beef. And if this be so, it becomes the duty of medical officers to provide some remedy, in the form of instruction to cooks on the philosophy of bread-making.

* The virtues of *saur-kraut* as an anti-scorbutic are well known, and although its smell (due to the presence of valerianic acid) is undoubtedly unpleasant, it deserves, in a sanitary point of view, a place in our army dietary as a condiment of much value.

soldier's dietary. Vinegar, as with salt and pepper, should never be wanting. Nor should the aromatic spices, cloves, ginger, and cinnamon be overlooked. They play an important and hygienic part in the domestic economy of the camp, and should not be restricted to the medicine chest of the surgeon.

But the virtue of food, however good, may all be destroyed by bad cooking. And this time-honored observation has led to the belief among many that while the Spirit of Goodness sends the food, the Spirit of Evil sends the cook! Be this as it may, the manner of preparing the food of soldiers is one of the most important of considerations, and as such deserves notice in this connection.

The French, who have systematized every thing down to the nicety of a mathematical proposition, insist in their army dietaries that the best possible preparation of animal food is in the form of soups. Roasts and stews with them only claim a secondary position. But in their field soups besides meat there are always vegetables introduced. We have then what New-Englanders call a *boiled dinner.* As a general rule it may be said that when soup is properly made, it furnishes us with all the nutritive elements of both flesh and vegetables contained in it. It presents to us animal juices in a state of solution, together with the mucilage of vegetables, and the sapid principles of both. But this highly concentrated form of nourishment should be qualified by consuming the now almost innutritious flesh and vegetables with which it has been made. We need the *bouilli,* or the woody fibre of the vegetable after partaking of the soup, because we need bulk as well as nourishment in our food. The intestinal canal must be distended as well as stimulated. Bread, also, should be eaten with it.

In making soups, good cooks say that the meat should be put into *cold* water, in quantity sufficient to be reduced *one-third* by boiling. The water should not at any time boil violently, but *simmer*, for from 4 to 5 hours, and no more must ever be added after the soup has begun to boil. Vegetables should be introduced for two purposes, viz.: to increase the nutritive qualities of the soup, and to flavor it. A knowledge of this fact will enable the mess-cooks to regulate suitably their proportions. Baked meats are more economical than broiled, or those roasted in the open air, both which lose by these last-named processes some of their nutritive qualities. All stews made of beef, mutton, or pork should be accompanied by appropriate vegetables and condiments.

Whenever practicable, fresh fruits should be allowed the men, in lieu of vegetables, but never in lieu of animal food.

As to beverages, coffee being a *regulation-drink*, and like water always to be had, nothing need be said on that score; but there are others which, under certain circumstances, are called for as a hygienic safeguard.

EDUCATED COOKS.

It is somewhat singular that, although the importance of good food to health is everywhere acknowledged, and the evils consequent upon ill-cooking are everywhere deplored, no means are yet adopted to remedy the latter by providing a corps of scientific cooks for our armies. The anathemas so constantly launched against the commissariat department for not providing the raw materials of good quality, might with great justice be distributed, in perhaps the largest measure, over the department of *kitchen and cooks.* Administrative vigilance limits its efforts to furnishing a due quantity of supplies, generally of an indifferent quality, and there rests. How the food is cooked, or whether it be cooked at all, is apparently a matter of perfect indifference to all in authority. The inconsistency manifested by such conduct is little short of criminal, for it is in every sense a neglect of one of the most efficient means for preserving the health of armies. In any other of the details of military service no similar degree of negligence would be tolerated. Were so many hundred pounds of powder to be issued to make so many thousand cartridges, no commander would rest satisfied with the report that the powder was dry, and of good quality; but he would insist upon knowing who were to make the cartridges—whether the workmen had the necessary tools given them, and whether they possessed the requisite skill. He certainly would not allow the unlearned to take part in the operation, except under the eye and direction of competent instructors.

Now some similar degree of vigilance is precisely what is needed in the culinary department of armies. We need, and we must have educated army cooks, in order to prevent disease, waste of food, and to extract the best possible good from it. Soldiers must be fed and nourished, as well as filled and distended by their rations. They are not anacondas, or ostriches, whose digestive organs can dispose of any thing that may be presented to their action. Hence boggy-bread, and leathery beans have killed more troops than bullets, and they will continue to do so, until some radical reform is introduced into regimental kitchens. It is idle to seek for probable causes of disease, in air, water, or earth, *outside* the camp, when so permanent and manifest a cause is assiduously at work *within*. The work of purification and prevention must begin *here*. The kitchen must be ennobled into an institution of science—of systematized intelligence, and of skilful adaptation of means to ends. In fact, cooks must be honored by an education in the chemistry of their own specialty. They should be taught the *how* and the *wherefore* of their art, and be elevated above the ignoble craft of scullions by a course of training calculated to win respect for them in the eyes of others.

Every company should have one *educated cook*, whose duty it should be to attend to nothing but the kitchen. He should be considered a non-combatant, and always retained as such. An assistant should be given him, but the cook alone should be responsible for the good dressing of the food.

Some such regulations as these would, if enforced, insure to each regiment a body of disciplined cooks calculated to promote in a very high degree the comfort of the men, and to preserve their health, by protecting them from the evil and insidious influences of bad cooking. And when the good results which may be thus secured at so cheap a cost are considered, it would seem as though it were only necessary to point them out in order to have instant measures taken to obtain them. It is certainly time that something were done in the matter. Humanity, no less than economy, is interested in the subject; for inexorable facts show that the dietary of troops is one of the chief avenues through which disease assails them, and that dietary, as all know, depends for its influence upon health, almost as much upon the mode in which it is prepared, as upon original qualities.

CHAPTER VIII.

THE CLOTHING.

THE clothing of soldiers, until recently, has never received that attention which its great importance deserves. The idea of its character, which obtained up to the middle almost of the present century, was evidently an inheritance of the past, and transmitted to us along with the legends of Wellington and Napoleon. A soldier, in those days, was a man in "brass and buckram" of formidable aspect, truly, but set in so thick a harness of padded cloth and leather, and so encumbered by the weight of arms, and of his clothing, as to labor under every possible disadvantage in a fight. Constrained in every effort by the *style* of his clothes, and oppressed on all sides by the unrelenting burthen which they and his arms imposed upon him, he could never be considered otherwise than an oppressed and fatigued man. Every thing in his equipment seemed calculated to obstruct freedom of motion and to impair his ability of performing muscular exertion. It seemed singular, indeed, that men whose duties called for the greatest agility, whose lives and whose successes depended upon the free use of every muscle, should by positive enactment be encased in a harness calculated to interfere with every extensive motion.

The terrible realization of this error was never forced upon European commanders until the French undertook the conquest of Algeria. There, the manifest advantage of lightly clad and armed troops over heavy ones was found to compensate almost for the deficiency in their military skill and discipline. Not alone on account of the climate, but also to remove every obstacle to agility which the French at once perceived was the strong point of all Arabic effectiveness, they proceeded to modify the dress of their army. An entire change of costume was the consequence of this observation. Every thing *heavy* and *constraining*, or *impeding* in any way the free movement of any muscle in either arm or leg, neck, shoulder, or back, was discarded. Loose pantaloons, and jackets, small collars, or none, light képis instead of heavy shakos, shoes in the place of boots, lighter rifles and muskets, took the place of the former heavy arms and accoutrements.

The world now recognizes the wisdom of this change, and is everywhere hastening to adopt it. Heavy, tight uniforms are giving place to light ones. The idea that either warmth or durability are dependent upon weight is exploded. We have, at last, made our exodus from this vestamental Jericho.

The first necessity of all dress is *warmth*, next to that, *lightness*. These two conditions are best fulfilled by *woollen* fabrics. Both the under and the outer garments of the soldier, therefore, should consist of this material. It is not necessary here to speak of the advantages of woollen over either cotton or linen. The world decided that ages ago.

UNDER GARMENTS.

Both in summer and in winter, in the tropics and under the pole, wearing flannel next to the skin has been found a protection to health. And except in extraordinary cases, and where some cutaneous idiosyncrasy forbids its use, troops should be made to wear it *night* and *day*. Where a whole waistcoat cannot be endured, a flannel *apron*, or *bandage*, covering the abdomen and loins, should be worn in like manner. Incipient diarrhœas and dysenteries are by this means often averted. Of the flannel bandage no praise, in fact, can be fulsome; it is the best friend of the soldier in all climates and seasons, and no one should ever go without it.

Besides the waistcoat, light flannel drawers should also be worn. These may be made of *cotton* flannel, which shrinks less, and for this purpose wears better than ordinary woollen flannel. Woollen socks are also necessary articles to health. But where any specific cause exists why they should not be worn, as by causing excessive perspiration and tenderness of the feet, thick *cotton* hose should be served out in their stead.

OUTER CLOTHING.

Inasmuch as regulation prescribes what this shall be, little opportunity is afforded us to say aught touching either the pantaloons, the jacket, or the overcoat. Of the necessity, as well as the advantage of their being loose, we have already spoken. But there is a subject connected with the uniform of soldiers, whose importance demands a passing word even at the hands of hygiene. That subject is its *color*, in relation both to warmth as well as conspicuousness.

Color plays an important part in the clothing of the soldier in two ways. First, as receiving and retaining more or less of the sun's rays, and being on that account *hotter*, and second as presenting better or worse marks for an enemy's aim. In relation to heat, it is well known that black or any dark colors are particularly absorbent of the sunlight, and consequently make very hot clothing. The manifest impropriety of selecting such colors for summer wear, unless, as in the zouave, the jacket is left open, becomes apparent to all. Such clothing are simply *sweltering* clothes, and harass the soldier unncessarily. The Arabs, daily exposed to the sun, wear a *white* bournouse, which, although made of woollen, is not in the least oppressive. A tight dark garment would be intolerable in their climate. But white cannot be kept clean, besides which it is too glaring to the eye, affords too good a mark to the enemy, and is therefore objectionable. The same reason applies to red.

.*Gray*, *buff*, or any neutral tint, presents us with the best requisites for a uniform.

But the second aspect under which color can be viewed in relation to uniforms, is that in which it presents itself as a mark for an enemy's aim. . The least possible thought upon the subject will convince us that all brilliant colors, red, orange, white, are, from their high reflective powers, visible at great distances, and consequently a fair mark for sharp-shooters. Therefore pickets, guards, and skirmishers should wear clothing of a more sober and neutral tint. Statistics declare that for every 12 men in *red* who are struck in an engagement, there are only 7 in *green*, and 5 in *gray*, thus showing the decided advantage of this last color over all others in point of immunity. These simple facts should be allowed to have more weight than they do in the uniforming of volunteer regiments, and surely, if color can in some degree prevent liability to bullet-wounds, and thus diminish the ratio of an army's mortality, hygiene does not transcend its province by calling attention to the fact.

The very small size of the képis and its closeness to the head, by forbidding all circulation, and keeping a heated cloth in contact with the skull, greatly predisposes to accidents by sunstroke. To prevent this, the so-called Havelock cap, or helmet of white linen, with a tail-piece shielding the entire neck, is a most desirable invention. This cap is worn by the British army in India, and proves an effectual protection against sunstroke. It should be at once adopted among our own troops.

Shoes with gaiters are the most desirable of all foot coverings for soldiers. They are lighter than boots, allow more freedom of motion to the ankle, and do not occupy so much room in the knapsack. The confined atmosphere of the boot, which under exposure to the sun becomes insufferably hot, keeping the foot in a vapor bath, and acting almost like a blister upon it, is entirely avoided in the shoe. The use of boots, in fact, should be prohibited to soldiers, as wearing them on a long march certainly impairs the soundness of men's feet. In summer, a white canvas gaiter should cover the shoe, as well to protect the foot from the sun, as to prevent the dust from entering it while marching.

CHAPTER IX.

ON THE PREVENTION OF DISEASE IN GENERAL, AND THE INDIVIDUAL PRESERVATION OF HEALTH.

ALTHOUGH what has been said in the foregoing chapters relates to the care of troops, and the maintenance of a better state of health among them in the various circumstances of their active life, I have still thought that it might be advisable to devote a special chapter to *the prevention of disease, and the individual preservation of health*, as furnishing suggestions for general and individual guidance under the ordinary necessities of a soldier's existence.

GENERAL GUIDANCE.

CLIMATE.

The sudden changes of climate to which soldiers are exposed in a campaign, are among the most important of the causes prejudicial to their health. When it is remembered also that climate does not so much depend upon latitude as upon the physical character of locality, it will be perceived that it is not necessary to transport troops many hundreds of miles in order to bring them under the influences of an entirely different clime. A change of a single degree in latitude may bring us where the nature of the locality, the soil, the character of the vegetation, and the prevailing winds, are as a foreign clime to our constitutions; while, even in the midst of a tropical climate a towering mountain will present us with zones of temperature varying from that of its base to that of the Arctic regions. Altitude is therefore a modifier of latitude. The climate of Vera Cruz and the *tierra caliente* is so entirely different from that of other places in the same latitude, but situate high above the level of the sea, that the inhabitants of these latter regions cannot enter what is to them, the *foreign* climate of the coast, without suffering from endemic fevers; and the same may be said of the inhabitants of the mountains bordering on the Roman campagna.

Observation shows that along the sea-coast and the borders of rivers, in the southerly part of temperate climates, the daily evaporation from the surface is productive of heavy dews, more or less laden with the products of decomposed vegetable matter. Where land-winds also habitually prevail, these products are dispersed over regions remote from the centre of their production. Contaminating effluvia are thus transported into the atmosphere of localities free from any internal sources of malaria.* Low grounds

* Dr. Ferguson was of opinion that the intermittent fever at Edinburgh was due to malarial poison wafted from Holland.—*Phil. Jour. Med. & Phys. Sci.*, No. 16, p. 374.

covered with vegetation, and bordering the sea-coast or the river-banks of southerly countries, whether they be actually dry or not, are always to be considered malarious regions, as towards new comers from the north.

Deep valleys or bottoms, where the diurnal variations in temperature between noon and night are noticed to be great, (from 15° to 30°,) may also be placed in the above category.

Situations at the foot of a mountain immediately rising from a low plain bordering the sea, are also objectionable.

Rains in all warm climates greatly increase the disparity of the temperature, and even in a single day may excite dysenteric affections. For this reason, the farther south we go the more protection we need against moisture, whether in the form of dew or rain.

The greatest liability to malarious poison (paludal intoxication) occurs when the equilibrium of the atmosphere is in a state of disturbance, as during some two hours after sunset, and two before sunrise. Within these intervals troops should not be exercised nor kept fasting. Breakfast should precede the performance of any morning duties, and supper should be eaten at sunset.

In order to acclimate an army with as little sickness as possible, it should enter the foreign clime at that season of the year which can most gradually introduce it to those extremes of heat or moisture, that mark its character. By doing this, all suddenness of transition is avoided, the clothing is not immediately obliged to be changed, nor the diet; the system gradually accommodates itself to the change in functions required, and the sickly season, when it does come, is met by constitutions already so much modified as to have lost much of their impressibility to endemic causes of disease. The ratio of sickness will always diminish in proportion to the degree of acclimation attained.

There are a number of duties occasionally devolving upon soldiers which, from the infrequency of their occurrence, are peculiarly distressing to those who undertake them. *Digging trenches, building bridges and causeways, making roads*, and the like, impose severe tasks upon soldiers. Yet these duties are at all times indispensable to the successful passage of an army through an enemy's country, and they must then be performed at any and every hazard. Their execution involves two of the most perilous conditions to health possible, in the form of great fatigue and exposure to terrene exhalations. Without some precautionary measures, this kind of duty affects the health of the soldier more than any other single cause, and when in particular the task is performed in a climate to which troops are not indigenous, visitations of disease may be speedily expected.

As a rule, therefore, whenever troops enter a foreign climate,* and until some considerable time

* I need hardly remark that our Northern troops, in passing now no farther south even than the lower Chesapeake, will, enter a climate entirely *foreign* to their constitutions, and that, too, at a season most likely to impress its character upon them. Thus,

has elapsed, they should not be called upon to make excavations, or greatly disturb the soil in parts not inhabited, or already brought under cultivation. If it becomes necessary to order such labor done, natives, when they can be employed, should undertake the task. For experience proves that in all alluvial districts the disturbance of the soil for the first time by the unacclimated, is sure to invite an attack of malarious fever. But where natives cannot be found to do the work, men should be selected who have come from adjoining districts, the chance of immunity always diminishing in the ratio of the distance of their usual habitations.*

Whenever troops are stationed either on the seaboard, or in malarious districts, their diet should be increased in quantity; overcoats should be worn at night, when on guard; and no out-door morning

New Englanders and New Yorkers will have traversed from five to eight degrees, and the men of the Middle and Western States from one to five degrees. From certain resemblances in soil and climate, it is probable that men bred in the great valleys of the Ohio and Mississippi (Missouri, Kentucky, Illinois, Indiana, and Ohio) will be less affected by these changes than those from our Northern seaboard States. It will be well to consider these things in garrisoning posts in the South, particularly in the low, alluvial regions bordering on the sea; or in the vicinity of lagoons, and the deltas of great rivers.

* Wherever great fatigue and continued exposure become inevitable in malarious districts, it might even be well to anticipate attacks of intermittent fever, by administering to those who are particularly exposed, a *one-grain* pill of the Sulph. Quinæ every morning fasting. M. Du Chaillu, the African traveller, assured me, that, by following this course, he had been enabled to traverse the most malarious intertropical regions with comparative impunity.

duties should be exacted of the men while fasting. Coffee should be dispensed to all who have returned wet and fatigued from mounting guard, or any other protracted exposure at night; the great object being to protect them against repressions of circulation due to the differences in temperature between midday and midnight.

Men, passing suddenly from a northern to a southern climate, suffer at first a sort of general erethism. Their systems are surcharged with heat, the blood is expanded, and there is fulness of the capillary circulation. If, now, they are exposed after nightfall to heavy dews and a temperature from 15° to 30° colder than the day, it is easy to divine what must happen to systems thus highly excited. "Cold," says Dr. Mosely, "is the cause of almost all the diseases in hot climates, to which climate alone is accessory." And cold acts upon the nervous system precisely as does the malarial poison, by depressing its tone, and lowering the functional activity of the large organs. Whenever soldiers have been thus circumstanced, and an incipient chill is felt, they should immediately, on returning to their quarters, lie down with additional covering over them, and endeavor to provoke a gentle perspiration. The sooner this is done, the less will be their liability to permanent disease. Every hour of omission aggravates the character of the disturbance, and that which was simply a slight chill, which a cup of hot coffee or a thick blanket could have dispelled, may soon pass into a form of obstinate and complicated fever.

When on guard at night, the best protection against sluggishness of the circulation is to keep the mind *active*. Be wide awake. The overcoat imparts no heat to the body—it only serves to retain that which is already there. The generation of it must come from within, and there is no better steam-engine for the human body than an active and thoroughly self-possessed mind, determined, by a concentration of all its energies, upon the task before it. Men exposed in the Arctic regions, never freeze to death so long as the mind is active, but the moment it goes asleep the body becomes fatally chilled. An active mind serves also to repel disease, and thus to preserve health. It is the conservator of the equilibrium of the vital forces, and regulates the measure of their activity.

After every exposure to wet, particularly at night, the men should be served with a ration of hot coffee, or ginger tea, and care should be had that they change themselves so as to sleep in dry clothes. And owing to the difficulty of drying clothing in a soldier's tent, each company should set apart a tent for this express purpose. The noisome smell, and the dangerous consequences to health, arising from keeping wet clothes saturated with organic emanations in an inhabited tent, cannot be exaggerated by any recital of ours. Proper drying quarters should, therefore, be provided.

Whenever an epidemic declares itself in camp or at a post, all ordinary precautions must be doubled. Active duties must be diminished in their duration, fatigues avoided, periods of guard-mounting lessened, and modifications made in the dietary, if deemed necessary by the medical officers. A sanitary squad, under the command of a surgeon's mate, should be organized, for the purpose of daily inspecting all tents, huts, barracks, kitchens, wells, and sinks. And a daily meeting of the staff and medical officers should be held, to hear reports upon the progress of the disease, to receive suggestions, and exchange opinions upon its origin, history, and character, and to promulgate orders for its speedy control and eradication.

Skirmishers are often absent at great distances from the camp, are scattered in small parties over a large extent of territory, and cannot, if wounded, immediately receive that medical relief which their case requires. They may be miles away from the main body, their own surgeons cannot be everywhere at hand to assist them, and hours may elapse before help can reach them. On a lone mountain-side, in a swamp or a thicket, the skirmisher may fall and perish, as hundreds have before him, undiscovered and unassisted.

"For want of timely aid
Thousands have died of medicable wounds."

In order to provide against these contingencies, there should, to each party of sixteen skirmishers, be given a small hospital knapsack containing field tourniquets, lint, and bandages, the carrier of which should be instructed how to use them.

INDIVIDUAL GUIDANCE.

The soldier, like the sailor, is proverbially careless of himself. His life, he appears to think, belongs to no one but the state, and he accordingly submits to whatever disposition of it she may make. But although it be true that the soldier does not own his *time*, and when under orders must always be ready, it does not follow that any one is master of his body. His person is still, within the limits of discipline, all his own. And his duties of personal self-preservation never cease but with life. It is his duty to take as good care of his health as he can; to be cleanly, temperate, industrious, and moral, because he is the custodian of his country's flag and of her honor; and must vindicate, by the uprightness of his character, his claim to be considered worthy of defending her.

With a view of assisting him to preserve his health, by pointing out the principal sources of danger to which he is exposed, the following suggestions have been compiled.

EXERCISE.

After violent exercise, avoid lying or sitting immediately, and in the shade, or with the wind at your back. Let your coat remain buttoned, or if previously open, then button it. Keep in motion for a little while, and out of the sun, gradually cooling off, and finishing by washing face, neck, hands, and arms in cold water. All who have witnessed the dangerous consequences that ever attend upon sudden checks of perspiration, whether through the instrumentality of air or the agency of cold water, will readily appreciate the language of the poet of health.

> "Hot from the field, indulge not yet your limbs
> In wish'd repose; nor court the fanning gale,
> Nor taste the spring. Oh! by the sacred tears
> Of widows, orphans, mothers, sisters, wives,
> Forbear. No other pestilence has driven
> Such myriads o'er the irremeable deep."

Drink not, then, while *hot* and wearied, on the march, from any stream, however tempting. Rinse your mouth, wash hands and face, but wait until you are cool before drinking, and then drink but little. In fact, the less water one drinks on a march through a strange country, the better. Change of water, more than any other single thing, induces derangements of the stomach and bowels, and to guard against it, every soldier should be furnished with a bottle of vinegar, a few drops of which will suffice to correct any brackishness or liminess of water.

But a far better thing is to fill the canteen before starting with half *coffee* and *water*,* *unsweetened*, which, when drunk cold on the march, is the best thirst-slaking and most refreshing beverage in the world. If coffee is not agreeable, tea answers just as well. Both these beverages are tonic, stimulant, and satisfying. Tea is more astringent than coffee, and

* The French troops depend entirely upon their *bidon* of *weak coffee* on the march, experience having convinced them that most waters are "flat, stale, and unprofitable," by the side of this.

for those disposed to looseness of bowels, is, on that account, preferable.

CLOTHING AND CLEANLINESS.

Without cleanliness of person no one can preserve good health. The skin being both a breathing as well as an eliminating organ, requires daily airing. It must be kept clean by friction as well as by frequent ablutions, but cleansing the skin avails little if the body-clothes are habitually soiled. For whatever is eliminated by the skin and absorbed by the clothing (being effete animal matter) is readily decomposed by the heat of the body, and becomes putrid. The necessity for changing the clothes and washing the body is therefore very apparent. It is a protection to health in the sense of being a purification of the body.

At least twice a week, in summer, the soldier, besides his daily morning ablutions of face, neck, hands, and feet, should wash his entire person. Soap should be used in the process. In winter, once a week may suffice.

He should never sleep at night in the flannel shirt, drawers, or socks worn during the day, but should exchange them for others of the same kind. If he is called in the night, he is just as ready with the shirt and drawers he has on, as he would have been with the others. At morning he should again resume the articles put off at night. By thus changing them morning and night, his body receives the benefit of an air-bath, and both his day and night garments have an opportunity to be aired, which should be done by *hanging them in the sun*, so as to allow a circulation of air around them. These may appear trifling things, but they are nevertheless of great importance to comfort and to health, as all will find who once adopt them. A pinch of salt is also a trifling thing, and yet the comfort and the benefit of a whole meal may depend upon it.

Flannels worn in this way need not be changed oftener than once a week, while, when worn night and day uninterruptedly, they would become foul and offensive in half that time.

But socks, whether woollen or cotton, should be changed twice a week. The perspiration of the feet renders them otherwise intolerably offensive, insomuch that the soldier's presence may become insufferable to his fellow-lodgers at night.

Avoid all sudden checks of perspiration. It is better to perspire than to shiver. So long as the skin is active and moist, there is little danger to health—

> "For while the effluence of the skin maintains
> Its native measure, the pleuritic spring
> Glides harmless by ; and Autumn, sick to death
> With sallow quartans, no contagion breathes."

When mounting guard at night in summer, it is better to wear an overcoat, even if compelled to keep it open, than to get chilled by going without it. A chill is the first stage of every kind of fever, and in southern latitudes is particularly to be dreaded.

Even if not so commanded by his superior officer,

the soldier should *always* wear flannel next the skin. But if it cannot possibly be endured, he should still wear a flannel *apron* over the stomach and abdomen, as a preventive to bowel complaints.

To protect himself against sunstroke, the Havelock cover to the cap should be worn, or, in the absence of this, a wet sponge, handkerchief, a few large leaves or grass, may be put in the cap. Abstinence from spirituous liquors will secure the soldier against predisposition to sunstroke, for it is found that the intemperate are usually the first victims.

No one should, on any account, lie in wet clothing. Blankets must be aired at morning, like every thing else that has been worn, and if *wet* should not be used.

When straw is used in tents for bedding, it must be daily turned, and when mouldy instantly thrown away.

Let there be kept up a good circulation of air throughout the night in the tent, by leaving the doorway open. If the rain come in on that side, shut it, and raise a part of the tent on the opposite side. But never sleep without some ventilating orifice. Good air is more essential than good food. A human being consumes about 18 pints of it per minute, or nearly two hogsheads and a half per hour; and air once *ex*pired is no longer fit to be *re*spired.

A small trench dug around the tent makes a good conduit for the rain, and prevents it from spreading over the surface of the ground; and the dryer the ground is in and about the tent, the better for the comfort and health of its occupants. For this purpose all grass should be plucked out as closely as possible, and not suffered to decay, as it will from the heat of bodies lying on it. As elsewhere said, the proper flooring for a tent is an India-rubber blanket. If the government does not furnish one, and the soldier can afford it, he should provide one for himself.

DIET AND DIGESTION.

Although the soldier's dietary is fixed by law, neither his appetite nor his digestion regulate themselves by it. They ever retain their own character, and suffer or flourish according to the degree of compatibility existing between them and his food. It is true that all men need good food and well cooked, but all men do not need the same quantity, nor to be fed the same number of times. Hence, rules of quantity and hours of eating are made to suit the average of mankind; and, within these rules, every individual must, by a proper study of his own temperament and wants, guide the daily conduct of his body.

As a general rule, sameness of diet, when long continued, weakens digestion in all men. Therefore let there be some variation daily, even if it only consists in omitting part or the whole of any article. The stomach will relish it all the better when it is again resumed. Thus, soup may be omitted at one dinner, and beef at another, and the beef may be eaten at evening, or, better still, the next morning, in lieu of a ration of pork. Always save any surplus beef and bread in your haversack against a time of need. It is more nourishing, more strengthening, and less cloying than pork, and when this latter happens to be the ration and you have no relish for it, the bread and beef will serve you a good turn. Never be afraid of good beef—it is the best foundation on which to build good health.

Avoid *fat* pork as much as possible in summer and in warm latitudes. It disposes to bowel complaints, and should never be made a staple article in any dietary. It should only be used to flavor other articles, or to fry with. Lean salt pork (hams, sides, or shoulders) is not open to the same objection.

Beans, unless thoroughly cooked, are only fit for horses. When half cooked they will provoke indigestion and diarrhœa in almost any one. The best preventive against them in such a state is to *let them alone*. All the vinegar and pepper you can put on, will not render them digestible. When sound and well cooked, however, they make an excellent *side* dish; but an entire meal should never be made of them. They should be subordinated to meat, bread, and potatoes. A little vinegar assists their solution, and pepper corrects their tendency to produce flatulence.

Eat your bread stale. It is lighter and more digestible; you will need less to satisfy you, and it will incommode you less, whatever the quantity eaten. Brown bread contains more nourishment than white, and is, besides, slightly laxative. Some of the strongest men in the world are fed on brown bread.

With rice, fat of some kind should be used as a flavorer. All mucilaginous articles of food—veal, pork, beans, and peas—should have a little vinegar added to them as a dressing, also pepper. In summer, vegetable acids, like vinegar or sorrel, are beneficial in small quantities.

Besides meat, vegetables are necessary to health. Any succulent roots, such as are put in soup, should be partaken of, but always as *side* dishes, and never as staples. Thus with beef, carrots or parsnips, either stewed or boiled, should be partaken of. Onions are also beneficial, and should be eaten. They are stimulating and somewhat medicinal.

Dried apples and peaches, when stewed, are desirable articles, and serve a good purpose in the system; being slightly laxative as well as refreshing. They should be flavored with a little ginger or clove, and kept as a valuable store to be used occasionally.

Ardent spirits are not necessary to health in the healthy. All authorities agree that their use is pernicious in warm latitudes, and the soldier is everywhere found to be better without them. Their place, properly speaking, is among hospital stores. There they should remain, and be dispensed only under the advice of medical officers. Abstinence from the use of spirits, when in the South, will be found a great preventive against diseases of the stomach and bowels.

PASSES.

The privilege of a pass is too often a privilege to the grave. The errors in diet, and the irregularities in bodily conduct, committed by soldiers when allowed to roam through a town, are so common, and so speedily visited by physical penalties, as to plainly indicate that this privilege is a dangerous favor to grant. It rarely happens that the hospitals do not attest, on the morrow, the consequences of this much sought-for dispensation. Lounging all day from shop to shop, eating sweets here, drinking spirits and acids there, gorging themselves with all manner of incompatible edibles, and drinking too often of spirits to excess, together with exposure to sun and dew; these are the parent causes of the mischief which so often attends upon "passes." Were men but to reflect a moment upon the line of conduct they so frequently pursue on these occasions, common sense would warn them of the accidents to health which they thus voluntarily court. It is in the excesses committed both in eating and drinking that lies the mischief. For, would soldiers only behave themselves out of the camp as in it; were they to eat at the same hours, and in no greater quantity, at the town table than at the mess table; would they avoid promiscuous drinking, and take spirits if they *will*, only with their holiday dinner—they would not find themselves groaning the next day under the doctor's care. Temperance in all things, imprudence in none, should be their rule and shield.

INDIGESTION.

Whenever an attack of indigestion is experienced, accompanied by nausea, make no attempt to check this latter with brandy or any other stimulant, until you have first aided the stomach in throwing off its offending contents; when this has been fully done by vomiting, then, and not till then, are stimulants allowable. Abstinence, rest, sleep, and small draughts of cold water, are better sedatives to an irritated stomach than either brandy or whiskey.

If diarrhœa * supervene, take no spirituous liquors to check it. Let the bowels first rid themselves of any offending matter; after which rest, extra warmth on the surface, so as to induce perspiration—an almost total abstinence from liquids, especially coffee, avoiding fat meat, beans, &c., will generally produce relief—within twenty-four hours. If pain and discharges still continue, report yourself on the sick list.

Constipation is never to be so much dreaded as diarrhœa, because it is always more or less under our control.† Diminishing the quantity of salt meat daily consumed, and increasing that of vegetables; avoiding an over use of pepper, drinking a tumbler of cold water fasting in the morning, soliciting nature at regular hours, and not omitting to attend to her calls when made; an observance of all these particu-

* Wherever there is an habitual disposition to looseness of bowels, much benefit is often derived from a simple abstinence from *liquids*. A *dry, unirritating diet,* has been known to produce an entire change of this condition and habit of the bowels.

† Neglected constipation is very apt to induce *piles*. In such cases, the best treatment is the application of a soft rag, wetted in cold water, to the fundament, immediately after an evacuation. Wash the parts, carefully push back any protruding pile, and on going to bed, lay the wet rag on, and keep it there all night.

lars will most generally afford relief. But if much headache accompany either constipation or diarrhœa, the proper course is to report yourself at once to the surgeon.

Taking cold, as it is commonly designated, is usually the result of unequal exposure of different portions of the body to the action of a low temperature. A man in a state of perspiration takes off his hat and fans himself, or remains in a current of air bareheaded, or removes his cravat; in a short time he discovers himself to be hoarse; he sneezes and gives other indications of a cold in the head. Another, under similar circumstances, exposes a larger surface of his person, and gets a more extensive cold. In either case, a state of partial congestion of the lining membrane of nose, throat, and possibly lungs, has happened. The capillary circulation, while in a state of great activity, has become suddenly arrested by the constricting effects of a low temperature upon the walls of its blood-vessels. What is the consequence? First, a slight chill; secondly, fever. Now, the remedy is a plain one, and consists in re-establishing the activity of the skin. First of all things, let the patient perspire, and the sooner he does so, the shorter will be the duration of the disorder. After the cold has "settled," it will be beyond his reach, and the surgeon will then need to interpose his skill. But until that time a man may, by early dieting, total abstinence from liquids of any kind for a day or two, and dressing warmly, recover himself without medication. It only requires immediate action, and perseverance in carrying out its details, to insure success. Napoleon used to treat his colds by fasting all day, and riding on horseback; two most excellent means for stimulating the circulation, and keeping up a constant moisture of the skin.

When the feet become tender from excessive perspiration—to prevent which, care should be had on a march to wash them night and morning in cold water,—bathing with spirits will harden and relieve them. This is usually done by pouring spirits into the boots when on. But a better and a cheaper remedy is good beef *suet*, which, when applied freely, checks inordinate perspiration, keeps them soft, and prevents cracks and chafings. Beef suet should always be included among a soldier's stores.

A veil, and a small bottle of camphorated oil for anointing exposed parts, will answer a good purpose to the soldier in southern latitudes, by protecting him at night from musquitoes, and those other innumerable insects that "mostly do congregate" there.

TREATMENT OF WOUNDS BEFORE THE ARRIVAL OF THE SURGEON.

As more or less time must always elapse between the reception of a wound, and the attendance of a surgeon, it will be well for every one to understand in what way temporary relief can always be afforded to the suffering.

Every soldier should carry about his person a large, stout handkerchief. This will, in an emergency, answer as a tourniquet, a bandage, or a sling for a wounded arm. A tourniquet is a strap made from any kind of material, and twisted tightly about a limb to check bleeding. A handkerchief, or a piece of rope, is the readiest thing out of which to improvise a *field-tourniquet.* In order to apply it, place the strap around the limb loosely, and tie it in a hard knot. Now bring the knot (which, if possible, should have a little pad of cloth under it) directly over the wound; thrust a stick between the strap and the limb on the side opposite to the wound, and twist it around and around until the bleeding stops, and then confine it.

Where the cut is large and gaping, first observe whether the bleeding is continuous or by intermittent jets; if the former, then *veins* alone are wounded, and the tourniquet should be applied *below* the wound, but as near its edge as possible. Where, on the contrary, the bleeding is by intermittent jets, then an artery is wounded, and the tourniquet should be applied *above* the wound; that is to say, *between* it and the heart. Never pour spirits of any kind upon a bleeding wound. It does no good, and only serves to irritate and to inflame it. Wash out all dirt from it with pure cold water, bring the edges as near together as you can, and apply the tourniquet as above directed.

Whenever any one has fainted from loss of blood, do not raise him up *suddenly* on any account. Raise his head slightly and slowly, if desirous to give him a restorative; but never raise his chest until he has fairly "come to," and breathes deeply. Before trying to restore him, it is wise first to check his bleeding, as during faintness the blood almost ceases flowing, and wounds can then be more easily attended to. In transporting him to the ambulance, and while in it, keep him horizontal, and free from sudden motion.

A wounded man is always thirsty, and then he needs, not spirits, but cold water; give him his choice in this particular, and you will see that *water*, *water*, is the unfailing request.

Whenever any penetrating wound of the chest is unaccompanied by external bleeding, and yet blood is coughed up, and suffocation seems at hand, keep the chest erect, fan the patient, cover the wound closely with a pad wet in cold water, and give him small sips of *spirit* and water.

Whenever joints are wounded, keep them in position, and free from motion, by wrapping a wet bandage tightly about them; and if any small, flat pieces of wood can be found, use them as *splints*, placing one on either side of the joint, and tightly bandaging it. In this way much pain may be avoided from muscular contraction, and even lockjaw be averted.

In all large wounds of the abdomen, particularly those involving protrusion of the bowels, keep the person lying down. Cover the wound, and place a bandage around the body to prevent motion of the bowels.

In wounds of the head, cold applications are always beneficial. Put on a wet pad. and a tight bandage over it.

Let the wounded always be handled carefully and tenderly, avoiding all suddenness of motion in transporting them, and making every provision for their comfort.

THE THROAT AND VOICE IN OFFICERS.

Officers, from a protracted use of the voice in an unnatural key and in a dusty atmosphere, are often troubled with irritation of the throat, which threatens serious damage to the voice. I have no doubt, also, that *smoking* induces a change in the follicles of the mucous membrane, whereby its secretions are greatly altered, and a pre-disposition to *roughness* and huskiness of voice is engendered. That pre-disposition can be eradicated only with the habit creating it. But during its prevalence, any extra effort to clear the voice, and to push it beyond its natural key will only result in producing chronic irritations of the throat. To avoid this, the voice should never be strained. By gradual efforts in the open air it can be greatly increased in volume. Should irritation, however, manifest itself, it will be well to frequently gargle the throat with cold water; or, if that be not sufficient, the addition of a few grains of tannin will impart an astringent character to it, generally desirable in relaxed states of those parts. A good preparation for those who are habitually troubled with irritation of the throat is, a solution of tannin in glycerine (two scruples to an ounce.) By painting the throat with this, which is neither irritating nor corrosive, great relief will often be obtained.

CHAPTER X.

ON HOSPITALS.

HOSPITALS are among the indispensable necessities of an army. Without them no force could be maintained in the field; for the gallant men who flock beneath the standard of their country would be demoralized, and dispersed after the first battle, by witnessing the unrelieved sufferings and the merciless sacrifice of their fellow-soldiers. If it be true, as Homer has sung, that

> " A good physician, skilled our wounds to heal,
> Is more than armies to the public weal,"

it is equally true that in an army the " good physician " is powerless to treat wounds and diseases without a hospital in which to place his patients.

But observation has shown that while hospitals are ever instituted to alleviate suffering and to promote good, they have, in too many instances, failed to accomplish either object, and on the contrary been instrumental in doing much harm. The bitter experience of Sir John Pringle in the campaigns of the British army during the last part of the eighteenth century led him to say that "hospitals are among the chief causes of mortality in armies." This truth has had, unfortunately, to be recognized even in our own day, but with this difference that we not only know whence comes this fearful mortality of hospitals, but have practically demonstrated the fact that it can be diminished by over *one-half*. In the general hospital at Scutari during the first part of the Crimean war, and which was very much over-crowded, *two* out of every *five* patients died, the mortality averaging about 42.7 per cent. on the admissions. In the *hospital-tents,* on the contrary, the mortality was only about half that, showing conclusively the advantage to be in favor of small-rooms, and fewer patients.

One of the principal causes of insalubrity in all hospitals is evidently the deterioration of the air due to the assembling of a large number of sick in any one apartment. In former days it was the fashion to have large wards, which, good enough in themselves, were yet entirely robbed of their advantages by overcrowding them with patients. Thus a writer, speaking of the Hotel Dieu, at Paris, in 1778, says, that in some wards there were from 500 to 800 patients, and in each of the large beds (52 inches wide) from 4 to 6 occupants! There was no classification of diseases either, but all were promiscuously commingled! It is needless to say that epidemics constantly raged in those wards, or that the mortality was exceedingly high. No amount of ventilation, in fact, short of tearing down the walls, could have relieved them of their pestiferous atmosphere.

The first and great requisite of all hospitals is a constant supply of pure, fresh air, brought directly into each ward, without passing through any room, corridor, or passage-way.

The sick require a more rapid change of air than the well. Their emanations, always more or less offensive, serve, when commingled in the atmosphere of a ward, greatly to depress the vital energies of each other; and thus a common retardation of recovery ensues, even if nothing worse happens. The offensiveness of the dejections in certain diseases, and of all discharging wounds in general, requires that military hospitals should beyond all others be well ventilated. And, indeed, unless this be done they are worse than useless, because they become simply foci of purulent infection to all their inmates. It would be far better to treat a wounded man out of doors, and with nothing but a blanket over him for a tent, than to subject him to an atmosphere which is very sure to develop gangrene. Besides *over-crowding*, which, as we have elsewhere seen, is so fruitful a source of increased mortality in hospitals, the external air may from various causes be vitiated, so as to produce analogous results. The position of the building with reference to sewers, marshes, stagnant streams, and the course of prevailing winds; or carelessness in the administration of its out-buildings, sinks, wash and cook houses, will all play an important part in determining the health and chances of recovery of its inmates. Miss Nightingale relates that in the hospital at Scutari the mortality rose

From	17.9 in Dec.
To	32.1 in Jan.
And	42.7 in Feb.

although the wards were not over-crowded, but *dead dogs* and *horses* had been lying for some time in its yard! At the Massachusetts General Hospital last year, gangrene developed itself immediately upon the opening of the mouth of a sewer in its vicinity. The disease had never been previously known there. In all hospitals situated in the populous parts of cities, the treatment of certain surgical diseases, is attended with much more uncertainty, and the percentage of recoveries is much smaller, than in suburban or rural hospitals. These facts show conclusively the immense influence which *locality* alone exercises upon the value of a hospital; for, unlike other and merely architectural defects, this one is irremediable.

The opinion is daily gaining ground that small *pavilion-hospitals* are better than large buildings with many stories. The number of human beings who can with safety inhabit a given area of ground is limited, and although stories upon stories may be built and tenanted, yet the law of nature is not thereby changed. As long ago as Hunter's day it was observed that the mortality in the *upper* wards, all other things being equal exceeded that of the lower ones; and the inference was thence drawn that there may be overcrowding as well by piling wards over each other, as by overfilling any one ward. In recently constructed European hospitals they have acted upon this suggestion by extending their area, and diminishing their altitude. This lightens the duties of the service very much, by bringing so many various rooms upon the same floor. Convalescents also can move about more easily, and having no high stair-cases either to descend or to climb, do not require so much personal attendance. In the cases of crippled men it becomes of great advantage, in allowing them to take short walks outside of the wards proper, to sun and air themselves in the grounds, and to be near their own quarters in case of faintness, or weariness.

Next to good locality, hospitals need abundance of *sunlight* in all their wards; and it is unnecessary to explain why, because of the universal knowledge of the benefits accruing to mind and body from the daily and direct influences of sunshine. Wards must be so constructed that the sun may be able to shine in them during some portion of the day.

Deficiency of space, for the numbers contained and the successful performance of the various hospital services, is another evil to be guarded against. While overcrowding relates more particularly to the condition of wards, deficiency of space includes the commingling in proximity of duties which, by reason of the noises produced by them, or the smells evolved, should be kept at a distance from the sick. Thus, the kitchen, the wash-rooms, and store-rooms should not be in contiguity to the wards. The smells of the one, and the noises of the other, would both disturb and distress patients. In the wards, beds should be at least *three* feet apart, so as to admit of a small stand or table between them.

Ventilation is, after all, the great desideratum in all hospitals. Plenty of air and a constant renewal of it, is what the sick must have. The size of the wards should be so regulated as to secure to each patient from 1,000 to 1,500 cubic feet of air, with ventilation adequate to supplying him with 60 cubic feet of fresh air per hour. This air, as before said, should come directly into the ward, and without first passing through any corridors, rooms, or passage-ways. Every such channel of ingress is more or less contaminating and therefore objectionable.

Beds.—The best beds for hospitals are *hair-mattrasses,* which are always smooth, soft, and springy. Straw is cold and hard, and wholly unfit for the sick to lie on. It is not advisable to place beds against dead walls, as more or less moisture is always emitted by them. The current of air flowing along their sides is cooler, denser, and therefore objectionable as a local atmosphere for the sick. Nor should beds be placed directly opposite to windows. Of these last there should be enough to have one window between every two beds.

Walls.—The walls of hospitals should be made of materials that are not absorbent; hard finish painted with some neutral tint is best. But in hospitals hastily constructed and intended only to be temporary, such precautions cannot always be taken.

They are often shanties or huts, hastily put up with boards and unsusceptible of more perfect finish. But even in such cases protection may be obtained by thoroughly washing them over, walls and ceiling, with some neutral tint. *White*-wash is too glaring to the eyes, and a mellower tint is better. The process should be occasionally repeated, taking advantage of an opportunity when the sick can be removed to another ward. It should never be done while they are in it.

Ceilings should be high, the higher the better; but never less than 12 feet. The bedsteads of iron; the furniture of hard wood, and the utensils of glass and earthen.

One nurse to every ten bedsteads, and one surgeon with two assistants to every fifty patients, seems about as little as will suffice.

The best size for wards on the score of cleanliness, ventilation, and facility of service is that containing about 20 beds.

List of Hospital and Field Supplies for the Sick and Wounded, as Recommended by the N. Y. Medical Relief Association.

1. BANDAGES.—Assortment and proportionate numbers of each variety required:—

1	dozen,	1	inch wide,		1	yard long.
2	dozen,	2	inches wide,		3	yards long.
2	"	2½	"	"	3	" "
1	"	3	"	"	4	" "
½	"	3½	"	"	5	" "
½	"	4	"	"	6	" "

2. Lint—Scraped and ravelled, in equal proportions.

3. Old linen and cotton cloth, without selvedge or seams, for compresses.

4. Ring pads and cushions.

5. Cotton batting and cotton wadding; fine flax and sponges.

6. Red flannel in the piece.

7. Bookbinders' boards for splints; pieces 18 by 4 inches.

8. Saddlers' silk for ligatures; wax, pins, and small pin-cushions.

9. Sewing needles, assorted in cases; linen thread, tape, and scissors.

10. Adhesive plaster, camel-hair pencils, oiled silk, oiled muslin, india-rubber and gutta percha cloths, in the piece.

11. Wrapping-paper.

12. Cotton shirts, drawers, and slippers.

13. Sheets, 4 feet wide and 6 feet long.

14. Bed-sacks, 3 feet wide and 6 feet long.

15. Pillow-sacks and towels.

16. Hospital knapsacks.

17. Field stretchers.

18. Eye-shades of green silk.

19. Lanterns.

20. Bed pans and urinals, metallic ones preferred.

21. Dressed sheep-skins.

FIELD HOSPITALS.

Field hospitals or *ambulances* are a part of the necessary equipment of armies. They are of two kinds, either *stationary* or *flying*. The permanent or stationary ambulance is located at some distance from the field of battle and out of harm's way; while the flying ambulance follows the regiment into battle, and affords provisional succor to the wounded until they can be transported to the stationary hospital.

As army regulations prescribe the details of arrangement for this class of hospitals, little need be said on the subject. Their temporary character, too, removes them from the necessity of those hygienic observances so indispensable in the construction of permanent hospitals.

The propriety of localizing the stationary ambulance near a stream of water, and of designating its location by a flag which can be plainly seen, will readily occur to every surgeon. What is chiefly wanted also, is a sufficient corps of *hospital-dressers*, to relieve the surgeon from all duty but that of operating.

In most of our volunteer regiments there is plainly an inadequacy of medical assistance. One surgeon and mate are not enough to perform successfully the ambulance service of a whole regiment. More *assistants* are needed, otherwise you will cripple the surgeon in times of pressing want by taking away his mate to attend the flying ambulance. This certainly is jeopardizing the lives of the wounded in a most reprehensible manner. "Considering how many young medical men there are who thirst for an opportunity as well to serve their country and humanity, as to perfect themselves in surgical knowledge, we cannot feel that the state could do our brave volunteers a more signal service than to enlarge the medical staff of our various regiments to an extent commensurate with what, it strikes us, must eventually become among the most prominent necessities of the medical service in our army. All will agree, at least, in the fact that the medical assistance hitherto provided to meet the exigencies of the terrible conflict that is impending, is not adequate to the probable necessities of the army, and that in no respect could greater service be rendered our regiments than by the organization and instruction of a sufficient number of good ambulance corps." *

* "*War and Medicine*," an article by the author, in the *American Medical Times* of May 4, 1861.

APPENDIX.

UNITED STATES ARMY REGULATIONS RELATING TO AMBULANCES AND HOSPITAL SUPPLIES.

The following are the decisions and recommendations contained in the Report of the Army Medical Board, (Jan. 19, 1860,) constituted by War Department Special Orders No. 195, current series, "to examine, select, and report such models" of ambulances "as it may think most suitable" for the Army; and to "examine the present standard supply table with reference to field service." They are published for the information of the Army:

1. That ambulance transportation ought to be furnished for 40 men per 1,000; 20 lying extended and 20 sitting.

2. That both two and four-wheeled ambulances are necessary for the hospital service.

3. That a two-wheeled ambulance is the best for the conveyance of dangerously sick or dangerously wounded men.

4. The Board being of opinion that both of the two-wheeled ambulances submitted to its inspection by Surgeon C. A. Finley and Assistant Surgeon R. H. Coolidge are well adapted to the purposes for which they were designed, and that their relative merits can only be determined by experiment, adopt both, and recommend that one of each pattern be sent to the respective Military Departments of Texas, New Mexico, Utah, California and Oregon, and two of each pattern to Fort Leavenworth, and that they be placed in service at the scenes of Indian hostilities, and on marches across the plains, in order that their practical advantages may be ascertained.

5. As the pattern of a four-wheeled ambulance designed by Surgeon Tripler, in the opinion of the Board, meets more fully the requirements of the service for the transportation of the slightly wounded, the slightly sick and convalescent, than any other pattern that has been submitted, the Board decide to adopt it, and recommend that three be constructed, and that one be sent to the Department of Texas, one to the Department of New Mexico, and one to Fort Leavenworth in the Department of the West, for trial in active service.

6. That of the two patterns of mattress frames presented for examination by Assistant Surgeon Coolidge, the one without the box be adopted for trial.

The service of Surgeon McDougall as a member of this Board being confined "to the consideration of the subject of a pattern ambulance only," and that duty having been performed, Surgeon McDougall was relieved, and returned to his post.

The Board, as originally constituted, then proceeded to the consideration of the amount and kind of transportation required for the sick and wounded and for hospital supplies; the allowance of hospital stewards, cooks, and nurses; and also the nature and extent of tent accommodation, for troops on marches and in campaigns against Indians, and for a state of war with a civilized enemy.

The following are the decisions and recommendations of the Board:

1st. The Board recommend that the following amount and kind of transportation for the sick and wounded be provided for troops on marches and in campaigns against Indians:

For commands of less than five companies, to each company, one two-wheeled ambulance.

For a battalion, of five companies, one four-wheeled and five two-wheeled ambulances.

For a regiment, two four-wheeled and ten two-wheeled ambulances.

2d. The Board, anxious to provide for the necessities and to secure the comfort of the sick and wounded soldiers to the fullest extent under all circumstances, recommend that the following schedule of transports for the sick and wounded and for hospital supplies, be adopted for a state of war with a civilized enemy:

For commands of less than three companies, one two-wheeled transport cart for hospital supplies, and to each company one two-wheeled ambulance.

For commands of more than three and less than five companies, two two-wheeled transport carts, and to each company one two-wheeled ambulance.

For a battalion of five companies, one four-wheeled ambulance, five two-wheeled ambulances, and two two-wheeled transport carts. For each additional company less than ten, one two-wheeled transport cart.

For a regiment, two four-wheeled ambulances, ten two-wheeled ambulances, and four two-wheeled transport carts.

And that the transport carts be made after the models of the two-wheeled ambulances, (their interior arrangement for the sick excepted,) and to have solid board flooring to the body.

The Board also resolved: That horse-litters be prepared and furnished to posts whence they may be required for service on ground not admitting the employment of two-wheeled carriages; said litters to be composed of a canvas bed similar to the present stretcher, and of two poles each sixteen feet long, to be made in sections, with head and foot pieces constructed to act as stretchers to keep the poles apart.

3d. The Board also recommend that the allowance of hospital attendants for a regiment in the field be, for one company, one steward, one nurse, and one cook; for each additional company, one nurse; and for commands of over five companies, one additional cook.

4th. The great size and weight of the present hospital tent render it objectionable in view of its transportation, and make it difficult and ofttimes impossible to pitch it on prairies and in high winds. The Board does therefore recommend that in future hospital tents be made according to the pattern of the present tent, and of the same material, but smaller, and having on one end a lapel so as to admit of two or more tents being joined and thrown into one with a continuous covering or roof.

The dimensions to be these: In length, 14 feet; in width, 15 feet; in height, (centre,) 11 feet, with a wall 4½ feet, and a "fly" of appropriate size. The ridge pole to be made in two sections after the present pattern; and to measure 14 feet when joined.

The Board contemplate that such a tent will accommodate from 8 to 10 patients comfortably.

The Board recommend the following allowance of tents for the sick, their attendants and hospital supplies:

Commands.	Hospital tents.	Sibley tents.	Common tents.
For one company................	..	1	1
For three companies............	1	1	1
For five companies.............	2	1	1
For seven companies............	2	1	1
For ten companies..............	3	1	1

The Board also recommends the adoption of a hospital knapsack, to be carried by a hospital orderly upon the march or in battle, who is habitually to follow the medical officer. The knapsack to be made of light wood; to be divided into four compartments or drawers, and to be covered with canvas after Colonel Buchanan's model knapsack, if that be adopted in the army. The purpose of this apparatus is to carry in an accessible shape such instruments, dressings, and medicines, as may be needed in an emergency on the march or in the field. The dimensions of the hospital knapsack to be those of the ordinary knapsack.

The Board respectfully request that one of each of the ambulances recommended for trial, be made under the immediate supervision of the officer by whom it was designed.

WASHINGTON, D. C.,
November 23, 1859.

STANDARD SUPPLY TABLE FOR GENERAL AND POST HOSPITALS.

Articles.	Quantities for one year for commands of—					Memoranda.
	From 100 to 200.	From 200 to 300.	From 300 to 400.	500 men.	1,000 men.	
MEDICINES.						
Acaciæ........lb.	2	4	6	8	16	
Acidi acetici........lb.	1/2	1	2	2 1/2	5	
" arseniosi........oz.	1/2	1	2	2 1/2	5	
" benzoici........oz.	1	2	3	4	8	
" citrici........lb.	1	2	3	4	8	
" muriatici........lb.	1/2	1	2	2 1/2	5	
" nitrici........lb.	1	2	3	4	8	
" sulphurici........lb.	1	2	3	4	8	
" " aromatici........lb.	1	2	3	4	8	
" tannici........oz.	2	4	6	8	16	
" tartarici........lb.	2	4	6	8	16	
Aetheris sulphurici loti........lb.	2	4	6	8	16	
Alcoholis........cong.	5	10	15	20	40	
Aloës........oz.	4	8	12	16	32	
Aluminis........lb.	1	2	3	4	8	
Ammoniaci........lb.	1/2	1	2	2 1/2	5	
Ammoniæ carbonatis........oz.	8	16	24	32	64	
" muriatis........lb.	1/2	1	2	2 1/2	5	

Anthemidis......lb.	1	2	3	4	8	
Antimonii et potass. tartratis......oz.	3	6	9	12	24	
Argenti nitratis (crystals)......oz.	1	2	3	4	8	
" " (fused)......oz.	1	2	3	4	8	
Arnicæ......lb.	1	2	3	4	8	
Assafœtidæ......oz.	4	8	12	16	32	
Bismuthi subnitratis......oz.	4	8	12	16	32	
Camphoræ......lb.	2	4	6	8	16	
Cardamomi......oz.	8	16	24	32	64	
Catechu......lb.	1/2	1	2	2 1/2	5	
Ceræ albæ......lb.	2	4	6	8	16	To be issued to posts where simple cerate cannot be sent without becoming rancid.
Cerati resinæ......lb.	2	4	6	8	16	
" simplicis......lb.	8	16	24	32	64	
" zinci carbonatis......lb.	2	4	6	8	16	
Chloroformi......lb.	1	2	3	4	8	
Collodii......oz.	2	4	6	8	16	
Copaibæ......lb.	5	10	15	20	40	
Creasoti......oz.	2	4	6	8	16	
Cretæ preparatæ......lb.	1	2	3	4	8	
Cupri sulphatis......oz.	2	4	6	8	16	
Emplastri adhæsivi......yds.	5	10	15	20	40	
" cantharidis......lb.	3	6	9	12	24	
" ferri......lb.	1	2	3	4	8	
" hydrargyri......lb.	1/2	1	2	2 1/2	5	
" ichthyocollæ......yds.	3	6	9	12	24	
Extracti belladonnæ......oz.	2	4	6	8	16	
" buchu fluidi......lb.	1	2	3	4	8	
" colchici acetici......oz.	1	2	3	4	8	

TABLE FOR GENERAL AND POST HOSPITALS—Continued.

Articles.	Quantities for one year for commands of—					Memoranda.
	From 100 to 200.	From 200 to 300.	From 300 to 400.	500 men.	1,000 men.	
Extracti colocynthidis comp.......oz.	8	16	24	32	64	
" colombæ fluidi...........lb.	1	2	3	4	8	
" conii...................oz.	1	2	3	4	8	
" cubebæ fluidi............lb.	1	2	3	4	8	
" gentianæ fluidi..........lb.	1	2	3	4	8	
" glycyrrhizæ.............lb.	6	12	18	24	48	
" hyoscyami ....oz.	2	4	6	8	16	
" ipecacuanhæ fluidi........lb.	1/2	1	2	2 1/2	5	
" piperis fluidi.............oz.	1	2	3	4	8	
" pruni virg. fluidi ....lb.	1	2	3	4	8	
" rhei fluidi...............lb.	1	2	3	4	8	
" sarsaparillæ fluidi.........lb.	2	4	6	8	16	
" senegæ fluidi............lb.	1/2	1	2	2 1/2	5	
" sennæ fluidi.............lb.	1	2	3	4	8	
" taraxaci fluidi...........lb.	1	2	3	4	8	
" valerianæ fluidi..........oz.	8	16	24	32	64	
" zingiberis fluidi..........lb.	1/2	1	2	2 1/2	5	
Ferri iodidi ....oz.	2	4	6	8	16	
" et quiniæ citratis...........oz.	4	8	12	16	32	
" sulphatis ....oz.	2	4	6	8	16	

Gambogiæ ....oz.	1/2	1	2	2 1/2	5
Guaiaci resinæ.....................lb.	1/2	1	2	2 1/2	5
Hydrargyri chloridi corr...........oz.	1/2	1	2	2 1/2	5
" " mitis..........lb.	1	2	3	4	8
" cum cretâ.............lb.	1/2	1	2	2 1/2	5
" iodidi ....oz.	1	2	3	4	8
" oxidi rubri............oz.	1	2	3	4	8
Iodinii ....oz.	2	4	6	8	16
Lini...............................lb.	4	8	12	16	32
Liquoris ammoniæ.................lb.	4	8	12	16	32
" ferri iodidi ....lb.	1	2	3	4	8
" potass. arsenitis ....oz.	2	4	6	8	16
" sodæ chlorinatæ ....bott.	3	6	9	12	24
" zinci chloridi ....bott.	3	6	9	12	24
Magnesiæ ....lb.	1/2	1	2	2 1/2	5
" sulphatis...............lb.	25	50	75	100	200
Massæ pil. hydrargyri ....oz.	8	16	24	32	64
Mellis despumati..................lb.	2	4	6	8	16
Morphiæ sulphatis................dr.	2	4	6	8	16
Myrrhæ............................lb.	1/2	1	2	2 1/2	5
Olei anisi ....oz.	1	2	3	4	8
" cajuputi ....oz.	1	2	3	4	8
" caryophilli..................oz.	1	2	3	4	8
" cinnamomi...................oz.	1	2	3	4	8
" menthæ piperitæ............oz.	2	4	6	8	16
" morrhuæ..................bott.	8	16	24	32	64
" olivæ......................bott.	8	16	24	32	64
" origani.....................oz.	4	8	12	16	32
" ricini..................qt. bott.	12	24	36	48	96
" terebinthinæ...........qt. bott.	4	8	12	16	32

TABLE FOR GENERAL AND POST HOSPITALS—Continued.

Articles.	Quantities for one year for commands of— From 100 to 200.	From 200 to 300.	From 300 to 400.	500 men.	1,000 men.	Memoranda.
Olei tiglii ....dr.	2	4	6	8	16	
Opii ....lb.	1/2	1	2	2 1/2	5	
Picis abietis........................lb.	1	2	3	4	8	
Plumbi acetatis........................lb.	1	2	3	4	8	
Potassæ acetatis........................lb.	1	2	3	4	8	
" bicarbonatis........................lb.	1	2	3	4	8	
" bitartratis ....lb.	2	4	6	8	16	
" chloratis ....lb.	1	2	3	4	8	
" nitratis ....lb.	1	2	3	4	8	
" sulphatis ....lb.	1/2	1	2	2 1/2	5	
Potasii cyanureti........................dr.	1	2	3	4	8	
" iodidi ....oz.	8	16	24	32	64	
Pruni virginianæ ....lb.	1/2	1	2	2 1/2	5	
Pulveris acaciæ ....lb.	2	4	6	8	16	
" capsici ....lb.	1	2	3	4	8	
" cinchonæ ....lb.	1	2	3	4	8	
" ferri ....oz.	2	4	6	8	16	
" " per sulphatis........................oz.	1	2	3	4	8	
" glycyrrhizæ........................oz.	4	8	12	16	32	
" ipecacuanhæ ....lb.	1/2	1	2	2 1/2	5	

Pulveris ipecacuanhæ et opii.......lb.	1/2	1	2	2 1/2	5
" jalapæ...................oz.	4	8	12	16	32
" lini.......................lb.	8	16	24	32	64
" opii.......................lb.	1/2	1	2	2 1/2	5
" rhei......................oz.	4	8	12	16	32
" sabinæ...................oz.	1	2	3	4	8
" sinapis nigræ............lb.	6	12	18	24	48
" ulmi......................lb.	2	4	6	8	16
Quassiæ...........................lb.	1/2	1	2	2 1/2	5
Quiniæ sulphatis..................oz.	10-20	20-40	30-60	40-80	80–160
Rhei...............................oz.	4	8	12	16	32
Sacchari...........................lb.	20	40	60	80	160
Saponis...........................lb.	4	8	12	16	32
Scillæ.............................oz.	4	8	12	16	32
Serpentariæ.......................lb.	1/2	1	2	2 1/2	5
Sodæ bicarbonatis................lb.	2	4	6	8	16
" boratis.....................lb.	1/2	1	2	2 1/2	5
" et potass. tartratis..........lb.	3	6	9	12	24
Spigeliæ..........................lb.	1/2	1	2	2 1/2	5
Spiritus ammon. aromatici........oz.	2	4	6	8	16
Spiritus ætheris compositi.........lb.	1/2	1	2	2 1/2	5
" " nitrici............lb.	2	4	6	8	16
" lavandulæ comp:.........lb.	1/2	1	2	2 1/2	5
" vini gallici.............bott	12	24	36	48	96
Strychniæ.........................dr.	1	2	3	4	8
Sulphuris loti.....................lb.	1	2	3	4	8
Syrupi scillæ......................lb.	3	6	9	12	24
Tincturæ aconiti radicis...........lb.	1	2	3	4	8
" digitalis.................oz.	4	8	12	16	32
" ergotæ (Dublin).........lb.	4	8	12	16	32

TABLE FOR GENERAL AND POST HOSPITALS—Continued.

Articles.	Quantities for one year for commands of—					Memoranda.
	From 100 to 200.	From 200 to 300.	From 300 to 400.	500 men.	1,000 men.	
Tincturæ ferri chloridi............lb.	1/2	1	2	2 1/2	5	
" veratri viridis...........oz.	4	8	12	16	32	
Unguenti hydrargyri...............lb.	1	2	3	4	8	
" " nitratis.......lb.	1/2	1	2	2 1/2	5	
Veratriæ ....dr.	1	2	3	4	8	
Vini colchici seminis..............lb.	1/2	1	2	2 1/2	5	
Zinci acetatis.....................oz.	1	2	3	4	8	
Zinci sulphatis....................oz.	1	2	3	4	8	
INSTRUMENTS.						
Buck's instrument for the throat...no.	1	1	1	1	1	
Cupping glasses or tins...........no.	12	12	18	18	24	
Dissecting.......................sets.	1	1	1	1	1	
Lancets, spring...................no.	1	1	2	2	4	Four extra fleams to each lancet.
" thumb ....no.	4	6	8	8	12	With cases.
Obstetrical......................sets.	1	1	1	1	1	
Pocket ....sets.	1	1	1	1	1	
Probangs.........................no.	6	6	6	6	6	
Pulleys ....sets.	1	1	1	1	1	

Scarificators	no.	2	2	2	3	4	
Splints (assorted)	sets.	1	1	1	1	2	
Stethoscopes	no.	1	1	1	1	1	
Stomach pump and case	no.	1	1	1	1	1	
Syringes, enema	no.	3	3	3	3	6	1 Davidson's; 1, 4-oz.; 1, 8-oz.
" penis, glass	no.	2	4	6	8	16	
" " metallic	no.	6	12	18	24	36	
" vagina	no.	3	3	3	3	6	Hard India rubber, 1; glass, 2.
Teeth extracting	sets.	1	1	1	1	2	
Tongue depressor (hinge)	no.	1	1	1	1	2	
Tourniquets, field	no.	4	4	6	6	10	
" spiral	no.	1	1	2	2	4	
Trusses, hernia	no.	3	6	9	12	24	
BOOKS.							
Anatomy	cop.	1	1	1	1	1	
Chemistry	cop.	1	1	1	1	1	
Dispensatory	cop.	1	1	1	1	1	
Medical Dictionary	cop.	1	1	1	1	1	
Medical Formulary	cop.	1	1	1	1	1	
" Jurisprudence and Toxicology	cop.	1	1	1	1	1	
" Practice	cop.	1	1	1	1	1	
Obstetricy	cop.	1	1	1	1	1	
Regulations for Med. Department	cop.	1	1	1	2	2	
Surgery	cop.	1	1	1	1	1	
Blank	no.	2	2	2	3	4	
Case	no.	1	1	1	1	1	
Meteorological Register	no.	1	1	1	1	1	

TABLE FOR GENERAL AND POST HOSPITALS—Continued.

Articles.	Quantities for one year for commands of— From 100 to 200.	From 200 to 300.	From 300 to 400.	500 men.	1,000 men.	Memoranda.
Order and Letter .... no.	1	1	1	1	1	
Prescription .... no.	1	1	1	1	1	
Register .... no.	1	1	1	1	1	
Requisitions, Returns, Reports of sick .... no.	1	1	1	1	1	
HOSPITAL STORES.						
Arrow root .... lb.	5	10	15	20	40	
Barley .... lb.	20	40	60	80	160	
Cinnamon .... lb.	1/2	1	2	2 1/2	5	
Cloves .... oz.	4	8	12	16	32	
Cocoa .... lb.	10	20	30	40	80	
Farina .... lb.	5	10	15	20	40	
Ginger, ground (Jamaica) .... lb.	1/2	1	2	2 1/2	5	
Nutmegs .... oz.	4	8	12	16	32	
Tea .... lb.	20	40	60	80	160	
Whiskey, bottles of .... doz.	2	4	6	8	16	
Wine, bottles of .... doz.	2	4	6	8	16	

BEDDING.						
Bed sacks ... no.	10	20	30	40	80	
Bedsteads, iron ... no.	6-10	12-20	18-30	24-40	48-80	
Blankets, woollen ... no.	10-20	20-40	30-60	40-80	80–160	
Coverlets ... no.	10	20	30	40	80	
Gutta percha cloth ... yds.	4	6	8	10	16	
Matresses ... no.	2	4	6	8	16	
Musquito bars ... no.	6-10	12-20	18-30	24-40	48-80	
Pillow cases ... no.	25	50	75	100	200	
" ticks ... no.	10	20	30	40	80	
Sheets ... no.	40	80	120	200	400	
FURNITURE, DRESSINGS, ETC.						
Bandages, suspensory ... no.	4	8	12	16	32	Assorted.
Binders' boards ... no.	4	6	8	12	16	18 inches by 4.
Corks, assorted ... doz.	12	24	36	48	96	
Cork screws ... no.	1	1	2	2	3	
Cotton batting ... lb.	1	2	3	4	8	
Cotton wadding ... lb.	1	2	3	4	8	
Flannel, red ... yds.	5	10	15	20	40	
Funnels, glass ... no.	1	1	2	2	4	
" tin ... no.	1	1	2	2	2	
Hatchets ... no.	1	1	2	2	2	
Hones (in wood) ... no.	1	1	1	1	1	4 inches by 1.
Ink powder ... papers.	2	2	3	3	4	
Inkstands ... no.	1	1	2	2	2	
Linen ... yds.	5	10	15	20	40	
Lint ... lb.	4	6	8	10	20	

TABLE FOR GENERAL AND POST HOSPITALS—Continued.

Articles.	Quantities for one year for commands of— From 100 to 200.	From 200 to 300.	From 300 to 400.	500 men.	1,000 men.	Memoranda.
Measures, graduated..............no.	3	3	4	6	6	
" tin..................sets.	1	1	1	1	1	
Medicine cups and glasses.........no.	3	6	9	12	24	2 cups to 1 glass.
Mills, coffee.....................no.	2	2	2	3	4	
Mortars and pestles, glass.........no.	1	1	2	2	2	
" " iron.........no.	1	1	1	1	1	
" " wedgewood...no.	1	2	2	3	3	
Muslin.........................yds.	25	50	75	100	200	
Needles, sewing..................no.	25	25	25	25	50	
Oiled silk or gutta percha tissue, or India rubber tissue..........yds.	4	6	6	8	12	
Pans, bed........................no.	2	2	3	4	5	
Paper envelopes..................no.	100	125	150	200	250	Assorted, 3 sizes. "Official business" printed on each.
Paper, filtering...............quires.	1/2	1	2	2	3	
" wrapping.............quires.	10	12	15	15	20	
" writing...............quires.	12	20	20	20	30	Foolscap, letter, and note—white; blue ruled.
Pencils, hair.....................no.	12	18	24	30	50	
" lead.....................no.	6	8	10	12	18	

Pens, steel......doz.	2	3	3	4	6	
Pill boxes......papers.	3	6	9	12	24	
" machine......no.	1	1	1	1	1	
Pins, assorted......papers.	2	4	6	8	16	
Quills......no.	25	25	50	50	50	
Rain guages......no.	1	1	1	1	1	
Razors......no.	1	1	1	1	1	
Razor strops......no.	1	1	1	1	2	
Scales and weights, apothecary's .sets.	1	1	2	2	2	
" " shop......sets.	1	1	1	1	1	
Scissors......no.	2	2	2	3	4	
Sheep skins, dressed......no.	4	6	8	10	12	
Silk, surgeon's......oz.	1/4	1/4	1/2	1/2	1	
" green......yds.	1/2	1	2	2 1/2	5	
Spatulas......no.	3	3	4	6	12	
Sponge......lb.	1/2	1/2	3/4	3/4	1	
Tape......pieces.	4	8	12	16	32	{ 1/4 woollen. { 3/4 cotton.
Thermometers and hygrometers...no.	2	2	2	2	2	
Thermometers......no.	1	1	1	1	1	
Thread, linen......oz.	4	4	6	6	8	
Tiles......no.	2	3	3	3	4	
Tow......lb.	1	2	2	3	5	
Towels......no.	20	30	50	75	150	
Twine......lb.	1	1	1 1/2	1 1/2	3	
Urinals......no.	2	3	5	6	10	
Vials, assorted......dozen.	6	12	18	24	48	
Wafers (1/2 oz. boxes)......no.	1	1	2	2	3	
Wax, sealing......sticks.	3	3	4	4	6	

Each Medical Officer will also be supplied with the following surgical instruments for his personal use, which he will retain in his immediate possession so long as he remains in the Army, and for the complete and serviceable condition of which at all times he will be held responsible:

AMPUTATING.

1 Capital Saw.
1 Metacarpal Saw.
1 Capital Amputating Knife.
1 Medium " "
1 Small " "
1 Large Catling.
1 Small "
1 Scalpel.
1 Tenaculum.
1 Artery Needle.
1 " Forceps.
1 Bone "
1 Spiral Tourniquet.
12 Surgeon's Needles.
1 Mahogany case, brass bound.
1 Gutta-percha Pouch.

TREPHINING.

2 Trephines.
1 Scalpel, with Raspitor.
1 Heys' Saw.
1 Elevator.
1 Brush.
1 Mahogany Case, brass bound.

EXSECTING.

1 Bone Forceps, Liston's.
2 Bone Forceps, sharp, assorted.
1 Bone forceps, for sequestra.
1 Chain Saw.
1 Chisel.
1 Gouge.
1 Lenticular Knife.
2 Spatulas, protecting.
1 Trephine, small crown.
1 Ecraseur.
1 Mahogany case, brass bound.
1 Gutta-percha Pouch.

GENERAL OPERATING.

1 Metacarpal Saw.
1 Trocar.
1 Ball Forceps.
1 Gullet "
1 Artery "
1 Dressing "
2 Scissors, straight and curved.
1 Artery Needle, with 4 points.
12 Surgeon's Needles.
1 Tourniquet.
1 Small Amputating Knife.
1 " Catling.
3 Bistouries.
1 Hernia Knife.
3 Scalpels.
1 Cataract Knife.
1 " Needle.
1 Tenaculum.
1 Double Hook.
6 Steel Bougies, silvered, double curve, Nos. 1 and 2, 3 and 4, 5 and 6, 7 and 8, 9 and 10, 11 and 12.
6 Wax Bougies, Nos. 2, 4, 6, 8, 10.
3 Silver Catheters, Nos. 3, 6, 9.
6 Gum-elastic Catheters, Nos. 1, 3, 5, 7, 9, 11.
2 Mahogany Cases, brass bound.
1 Gutta-percha Pouch.

POCKET.

1 Large Scalpel.
1 Small "
1 Artery Forceps.
1 Bull-dog "
1 Curved "
1 Dressing "

1 Needle.	1 Exploring Needle.
1 Sharp-pointed Bistoury.	1 Exploring Trocar.
1 Probe-pointed "	1 Seton Needle.
1 Long Probe-pointed Bistoury.	1 Spatula.
1 Straight Scissors.	2 Probes.
1 Knee "	1 Director.
1 Flat-curved Scissors.	1 Double Canula.
1 Gum Lancet.	1 Comp'd Silver Catheter.
1 Tenaculum.	6 Surgeon's Needles.
1 Tenotomy Knife.	1 Artery Needle.
1 Abscess Lancet.	1 Morocco Case.

1 Leather Trunk.

To each General and Post Hospital, one ounce of *brominium*, with printed directions for preparing and administering Bibron's antidote to the poison of *serpents.* Also one bottle of *liquor ferri per sulphatis*, and one bottle of *liquor ammoniæ*, in equal proportions, with printed directions for preparing speedily and for administering the *hydrated sesqui-oxide of iron*, as an antidote to poisoning by *arsenic.*

If the following articles of Hospital Furniture cannot be obtained with the hospital fund, they may be procured from a quartermaster or medical disbursing officer, by special requisition:

ARTICLES.

Basins, wash.	Mugs.
Bowls.	Pans, frying.
Brushes.	" sauce.
Buckets.	Pitchers.
Candlesticks.	Plates and Dishes.
Clothes Lines.	Pots, chamber and chair.
Cups.	" coffee and tea.
Dippers and Ladles.	Sadirons.
Graters.	Shovels, fire.
Gridirons.	Snuffers.
Kettles, tea.	Spoons.
Knives and forks.	Tongs and Pokers.
Lamps and Lanterns.	Tumblers.
Locks and Keys.	Woodsaws.

STANDARD SUPPLY TABLE FOR FIELD SERVICE.

ARTICLES.	Quantities. Reg't 3 mos.	Bat. 3 mos.	Comp. 3 mos.	MEMORANDA.
MEDICINES.				
Acidi acetici......lb.	1	1/2	1/2	
" sulphurici aromatici......lb.	1	1/2	1/4	
" tannici......oz.	2	1	1	
Alcoholis......cong.	2	1	1/2	
Aluminis......lb.	1	1/2	1/4	
Ammoniæ carbonatis......oz.	16	8	4	
Antimonii et potass. tartratis......oz.	2	1	1	
Argenti nitratis (crystals)......oz.	2	1	1/2	
" " (fused)......oz.	2	1	1/2	
Brominii......oz.	1	1	1	
Camphoræ......lb.	4	2	1	
Ceræ albæ......oz.	2	2	1	
Cerati resinæ......lb.	2	1	1/2	
" simplicis......lb.	8	4	2	
Chloroformi......lb.	2	1	1	
Copaibæ......lb.	2	1	1/2	
Creasoti......oz.	2	1	1	
Cupri sulphatis......oz.	4	2	1	
Emplastri adhæsivi......yds.	10	5	3	
" cantharidis......lb.	4	2	1	

Emplastri ichthyocollæ ....yds.	10	5	3
Extracti belladonnæ..............oz.	1	1	1
" buchu fluidi..............lb.	1	1/2	1/4
" colchici acetici...........oz.	2	1	1
" colocynthidis comp.......oz.	16	8	4
" glycyrrhizæ..............lb.	2	1	1/2
" rhei fluidi...............lb.	2	1	1/2
" senegæ fluidi.............oz	8	4	4
" sennæ fluidi..............lb.	2	1	1/2
Ferri per sulphatis................oz.	4	2	1
Hydrargyri chloridi corrosivi ......oz.	1/2	1/2	1/2
" " mitis..........lb.	2	1	1/2
Iodinii ....oz.	4	2	1
Liquoris ammoniæ................lb.	4	2	1
" potass. arsenitis ....oz.	4	2	1
Magnesiæ sulphatis...............lb.	20	10	5
Massæ pil. hydrargyri ....oz.	16	8	4
Morphiæ sulphatis................dr.	4	2	1
Olei caryophilli ....oz.	1	1	1
" menthæ piperitæ.............oz.	2	1	1
" olivæ......................bott.	8	4	2
" ricini...................qt. bott.	12	6	3
" terebinthinæ............qt. bott.	8	4	2
" tiglii.......................dr.	2	1	1
Pilul. cathartic. comp. (U. S.)....doz.	8	4	2
" opii (U. S.)................doz.	8	4	2
" quiniæ sulphatis (3 grs.).....oz.	8	4	2
Plumbi acetatis...................lb.	2	1	1/2
Potassæ bicarbonatis..............lb.	1	1/2	1/4
" chloratis................lb.	2	1	1/2

TABLE FOR FIELD SERVICE—Continued.

Articles.	Quantities.			Memoranda.
	Reg't 3 mos.	Bat. 3 mos.	Comp. 3 mos.	
Potasse nitratis ....lb.	1	1/2	1/4	
Potasii cyanureti....................dr.	1	1	1	
" iodidi ....oz.	8	4	2	
Pulveris acaciæ ....lb.	4	2	1	
" capsici ....lb.	1/2	1/4	1/4	
" ipecacuanhæ ....lb.	1	1/2	1/4	
" " et opii........oz.	8	4	4	
" lini........................lb.	16	8	4	
" opii........................lb.	2	1	1/2	
" rhei ....lb.	1/2	1/4	1/4	
" sinapis nigræ..............lb.	12	6	3	
Quiniæ sulphatis....................oz.	24	12	6	
Sacchari..........................lb.	10	5	2	
Saponis..........................lb.	8	4	2	
Sodæ bicarbonatis ....lb.	1	1/2	1/2	
Spiritus ammoniæ aromatici ......oz.	4	2	2	
" ætheris comp..............lb.	1	1/2	1/2	
" " nitrici............lb.	2	1	1/2	
" vini gallici ....bott.	24	12	6	
Strychniæ..........................dr.	1	1	1	
Tincturæ aconiti radicis............lb.	1	1/2	1/4	
" ferri chloridi............lb.	1	1/2	1/4	

Tincturæ opii......................oz.	16	8	6	
" veratri viridis...........oz.	8	4	2	
Unguenti hydrargyri..............lb.	1	1/2	1/4	
" " nitratis.......lb.	1/2	1/4	1/4	
Zinci acetatis......................oz.	2	1	1	
Zinci sulphatis....................oz.	2	1	1	
INSTRUMENTS.				
Buck's instrument for the throat...no.	1	1	1	
Cupping glasses and tins ....no.	16	8	4	Half glass, half tin.
Lancets, spring...................no.	1	1	1	
" thumb (with cases) ......no.	6	4	2	
Pocket ....sets.	1	1	1	
Probangs, whalebone.............no.	12	6	2	
Scarificators ....no.	4	2	1	
Splints (major) ....sets.	1	1	1	
Stomach pump and case...........no	1	1	1	
Syringes, enema...................no.	4	2	1	1 Davidson's; 1 hard rubber, 6 oz.
" penis, glass..............no.	8	4	2	
" " India rubber......no.	8	4	2	
Teeth extracting.................sets.	1	1	1	
Tongue depressor (hinge).........no.	1	1	1	
Tourniquets, field.................no.	8	4	2	
" spiral................no.	2	2	1	
Trusses, hernia ....no.	6	3	2	
BOOKS.				
Anatomy (surgical)..............cop.	1	1	1	

TABLE FOR FIELD SERVICE—Continued.

Articles.	Quantities.			Memoranda.
	Reg't 3 mos.	Bat. 3 mos.	Comp. 3 mos.	
Medical Practice ....cop.	1	1	1	
Regulations for Med. Department.cop.	1	1	1	
Surgery (operative).............cop.	1	1	1	
Thompson's Conspectus..........cop.	1	1	1	
Blank..........................no.	4	4	4	
HOSPITAL STORES.				
Arrow root......................lb.	10	5	3	
Candles (sperm).................lb.	2	1	1	
Farina..........................lb.	10	5	3	
Ginger (fluid extract)............lb.	1	1/2	1/4	
Nutmegs ....oz.	8	4	2	
Tea.............................lb.	30	15	7	
Whiskey, bottles of.............doz.	2	1	1/2	
BEDDING.				
Blankets, woollen ....no.	20-40	10-20	10	Brown.
Blanket cases ....no.	1 for	10 bla	nkets.	Of canvas, after pattern.
Gutta-percha cloth...............yds.	8	4	2	
" " bed covers.........no.	8	4	2	So constructed as to form, when united, a continuous spread or covering.

Musquito bars.....................no.	12	6	4	
FURNITURE AND DRESSINGS.				
Bandages, roller, assorted........doz.	14	7	4	
" suspensory, assorted....no.	12	6	4	
Binders' boards.....................no.	18	9	5	18 inches by 4.
Buckets, leather.....................no.	4	2	2	BANDAGES.
Corks, assorted.....................doz.	12	6	3	1 dozen, 1 inch wide, 1 yard long.
Corkscrews.........................no.	2	1	1	2 " 2 " 3 "
Cotton batting.......................lb.	2	1	1/2	2 " 2 1/2 " 3 "
" wadding.....................lb.	2	1	1/2	1 " 3 " 4 "
Flannel, red.........................yds.	5	3	2	1/2 " 3 1/2 " 5 "
Hatchets.............................no.	2	1	1	1/2 " 4 " 6 "
Hones.................................no.	1	1	1	4 inches by 1, in wood.
Ink, 2-ounce bottles...............no.	12	6	3	
Knapsack, hospital.................no.	..	..	..	According to pattern.
Lanterns.............................no.	4	2	1	
Lint...................................lb.	8	4	2	
Litters and stretchers, hand.......no.	..	..	..	} According to pattern.
" horse.....................no.	..	..	..	}
Measures, graduated, assorted.....no.	4	2	2	6 oz., 2 oz., minim.
Medicine chests.....................no.	..	..	..	
" cups and glasses..........no.	6	3	2	2 cups to one glass.
" panniers.................no.	..	..	..	
Mess chests.........................no.	..	..	..	See note.
Mills, coffee.........................no.	2	1	1	
Mortars and pestles, wedgewood...no.	2	1	1	Small.
Muslin...............................yds.	20	10	5	
Needles, sewing.....................no.	25	25	25	Assorted, in a case.

TABLE FOR FIELD SERVICE—Continued.

Articles.	Quantities. Reg't 3 mos.	Bat. 3 mos.	Comp. 3 mos.	Memoranda.
Oiled silk or gutta-percha tissue, or India-rubber tissue..........yds.	8	4	2	
Pans, bed..........no.	2	1	1	Of hard India-rubber or other material. Shovel.
Paper envelopes, assorted..........no.	100	50	25	50 letter, 25 note, 25 large. "Official business" printed on each.
Paper, wrapping..........quires.	6	3	1	
" writing..........quires.	12	6	3	2 foolscap, 6 letter, 4 note, white; blue ruled.
Pencils, hair..........no.	24	12	6	
" lead..........no.	12	6	3	Of Faber's make, No. 2.
Pens, steel..........doz.	4	2	1	
Pill-boxes (wood)..........papers.	2	1	1	
" (tin)..........no.	6	6	6	
Pins, assorted..........papers.	4	2	2	Large and medium.
Razors..........no.	1	1	1	
Razor strops..........no.	1	1	1	
Scales and weights, apothecary's .sets.	1	1	1	
Scissors..........no.	4	2	2	
Sheep-skins, dressed..........no.	4	2	1	
Silk, surgeon's..........oz.	1/2	1/4	1/4	
" green..........yds.	1	1/2	1/2	

Spatulas........................no.	6	3	2	
Sponge (washed)..................lb.	1	1/2	1/4	
Tape........................pieces.	4	2	1	
Thread, linen...................oz.	2	1	1	
Tiles ....no.	2	1	1	
Towels ....no.	40	20	10	
Twine ....lb.	1/2	1/4	1/4	
Urinals.........................no.	4	2	1	
Vials, assorted..............dozen.	4	2	1	1 oz. and 2 oz.
Wafers (1/2 oz. boxes)..........no.	1	1	1	
Wax, sealing.................sticks.	2	1	1	

NOTE.—Furniture of Mess Chest.

8 Basins, tin.
2 Boxes, pepper and salt.
6 Cups, tin.
4 Canisters, (for tea, coffee, sugar, and butter.)
2 Dippers and ladles.
1 Grater.
1 Gridiron.
1 Kettle, tea, iron.
12 Knives and forks.
6 Mugs, (Britannia, 1/2 pint.)
1 Pan, frying.
1 Pan, sauce.
8 Plates (6) and dishes (2), tin.
1 Pot, iron.
2 Pots, coffee and tea, tin.
12 Spoons, iron, (table [6] and tea [2].)
1 Tray, tin.
6 Tumblers, tin.

The above report and proposed supply tables are approved and adopted, and will be observed by all concerned, and existing General Regulations are modified so as to conform to the same. The tables contain all the articles to be purchased by medical purveyors, except on the orders of the Surgeon-General; but any less quantity may be required, or any article omitted, at the discretion of the medical officer.

The transfer of the surgical instruments issued to each medical officer for his personal use, is positively forbidden. These instruments will be accounted for to the Surgeon-General on the 31st day of December annually: in a special return, in which the true condition of each must be stated; and if any be lost or damaged, a report of the facts and circumstances attending such loss or damage must be given.

The Quartermaster Department will cause ambulances of each pattern to be constructed without unnecessary delay, as follows: one at Philadelphia under the supervision of Surgeon C. A. Finley, one at Cincinnati under Surgeon C. S. Tripler, and one at Washington, D. C., under Assistant-Surgeon R. H. Coolidge. He will then cause seven of each of the two-wheeled, and three of the four-wheeled ambulances to be constructed after these as models, and distributed as designated by the Board, for trial in active service according to the recommendation of the same, under direction of the several Department Commanders.

BY ORDER OF THE SECRETARY OF WAR:

S. COOPER,
Adjutant-General.

OFFICIAL:

Assistant Adjutant-General.

AUSCULTATORY PERCUSSION CHART.

THORAX.

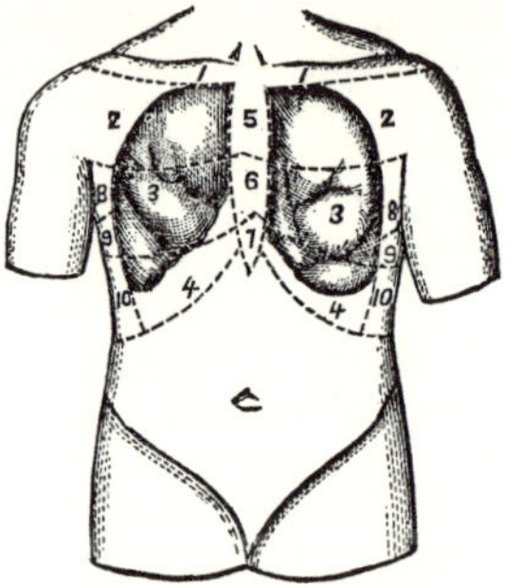

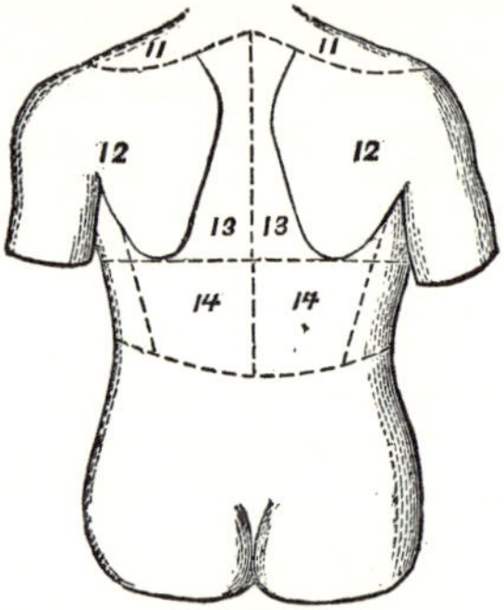

ANTERIOR.

1. 1. Clavicular Regions.
2. 2. Sub-Clavian.
3. 3. Mammary.
4. 4. Infra-Mammary.
5. 6. The Sternal.
7. The Lower Sternal.

LATERAL.

8. 8. Axillary Regions.
9. 9. Lateral do.
10. 10. Lower Lateral.

POSTERIOR.

11. 11. Acromial Regions.
12. 12. Scapular do.
13. 13. Inter-Scapular do.
14. 14. Dorsal.

ABDOMEN.

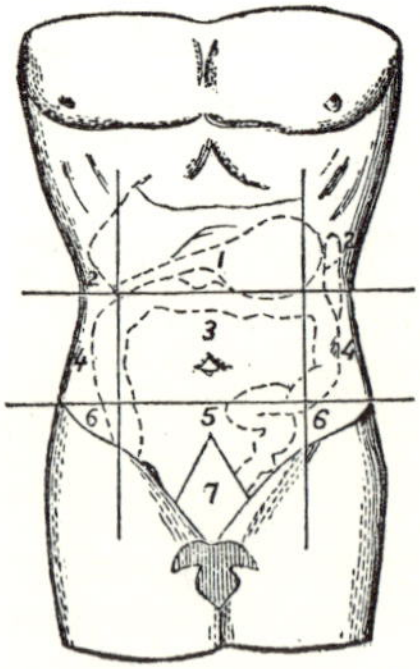

1. Epigastric.
2. 2. Right and Left Hypochondriac.
3. Umbilical.
4. 4. Right and Left Iliac.
5. Hypogastric.
6. 6. Right and Left Inguinal.
7. Pubic.

MANUAL OF INSTRUCTIONS

FOR

MILITARY SURGEONS,

ON THE

EXAMINATION OF RECRUITS AND DISCHARGE OF SOLDIERS.

With an Appendix,

CONTAINING THE OFFICIAL REGULATIONS OF THE PROVOST-MARSHAL GENERAL'S BUREAU, AND THOSE FOR THE FORMATION OF THE INVALID CORPS, ETC., ETC.

PREPARED AT THE REQUEST OF THE UNITED STATES SANITARY COMMISSION,

BY

JOHN ORDRONAUX, M. D.,

PROFESSOR OF MEDICAL JURISPRUDENCE IN COLUMBIA COLLEGE, NEW YORK.

NEW YORK:

D. VAN NOSTRAND, 192 BROADWAY.

LONDON: TRÜBNER & CO.

1863.

C. A. ALVORD, STEREOTYPER AND PRINTER.

DEDICATED

TO

BRIGADIER-GENERAL WILLIAM A. HAMMOND,

SURGEON-GENERAL, UNITED STATES ARMY.

PREFACE.

The accompanying manual was prepared at the request of the United States Sanitary Commission, as a contribution to *Military Medical Jurisprudence*, a department whose importance is second to none in the domain of military medicine. And while aware that it would amply justify an enlarged treatise of its own, the Commission, in accordance with their usual practice in issuing medical monographs, have selected this as the most condensed and practically useful form, in which to present surgeons with a complete aide-memoire upon the subject of which it specially treats.

In undertaking the duty of its preparation, the single point kept in view, therefore, has been that of embodying in a form of succinct exposition, the whole of the vast and complex subject of physical disabilities in their relation to the military service. It has been my aim, at the outset, to be brief without being obscure—to omit nothing of indispensable, or even ordinary importance—and to draw my materials from the best accredited sources of information, and the highest authorities of the old world, because of the ages of experience possessed by European nations, and the large amount of knowledge preserved in their medical annals upon this branch of military hygiene.

Selecting France and Prussia as the representative military nations of Europe, I have followed and adopted, as closely as possible, their codes of instruction on the subjects of the enlistment or discharge of soldiers. The Prussian code of 1858, entitled as follows:

"*Instruktion für Militair-Aerzte zur Untersuchung und Beurtheilung der Diensbranchbarkeit oder Unbranchbarkeit Militairpflichtiger Rekruten resp. Soldaten, so wie zur Beurtheilung der Invaliditat im Dienst befindlicher oder entlassener versorgungsberechtighter Soldaten.*" *Berlin den* 9 *Dez.* 1858, *per Dr. Grimm, General-Stab-Arzt der Armee und Chef des Militair-Medizinal-Wesens,*

contains only thirty-six pages, while the French code of 1862, entitled,

"*Instructions pour les officiers de Santé sur les Infirmités ou Maladies qui rendent impropre au service Militaire.*" *Approuvé par le Maréchal de France, Ministre Secrétaire d'Etat de la Guerre, le* 2 *Avril* 1862, *d'apres la proposition du Conseil de Santé des Armees,*

contains one hundred and forty-five pages. This latter being not only the most recent, but also the most ample and exhaustive, was accordingly selected as the foundation of my manual. With the exception of the introduction, and the leading sections treating of generalities, which immediately follow it, the manual is, for the most part, a *free* translation of the French code. It was at first intended to have translated it literally, and to have thus adopted it without alteration, but on discussing the subject in a committee of medical gentlemen, it was deemed advisable, and as likely better to meet the wants of American surgeons, to entirely reconstruct certain parts, and to alter so many others in various ways, as to render it more of a paraphrase than, strictly speaking, a translation. The diffuse and discursive style so common to French writers, together with other idiomatic and professional peculiarities which need not here be mentioned, all conspired to justify the wisdom of this decision.

Brief notes have also been added, whenever the subject under discussion seemed to require further illustration, and, if few in number, both their paucity and brevity must be charged to the single desire, expressed at the outset, of making the work a simple manual, rather than an expanded treatise like those of Coche, Marshall, or Fallot.

In the preparation of a work of this kind, involving as it does a special and accurate knowledge of so many departments of medical science, no single, unaided mind could safely venture to trust to its own resources. And I am happy in this connection, therefore, to acknowledge my great and lasting obligations to Dr. William H. Van Buren, Professor of Anatomy, in the University of the city of New York, for his patient and critical revision of my manuscript, and the many valuable suggestions offered by him in the course of its preparation. Nor am I the less under obligations of an equally lasting character to Dr. Cornelius R. Agnew, one of the surgeons of the New York Eye Infirmary, who has not simply revised, but largely reconstructed the section on Diseases of the Eye.

Many passages in the manual bear an impress of obscurity,

which, it is almost needless to say, has been purposely given them, in order not to furnish any instruments of deception to those, who might seek here for assistance in accomplishing themselves in the art of malingering. While keeping this possibility constantly in view, it is believed that nothing of real importance to surgeons has been omitted.

I have embodied in the form of an appendix, the code of instructions relating to the United States Army, adopted by the Board of Medical Officers, convened in Washington for that purpose, on the 15th of April, 1863, to which I have further added the Regulations governing the formation of our Invalid Corps; the Prussian list of disqualifying diseases, and the Regulations governing the formation of their Invalid Corps.

The following pages are now committed to the candid judgment and impartial criticism of the profession, in the hope that they will both subserve the interests of those for whose benefit they were written, and be found worthy of the subject they are intended to illustrate.

J. O.

NEW YORK, *June*, 1863.

TABLE OF CONTENTS.

INTRODUCTION.

SECTION PAGE

I.—Duties of Medical Examiners; Instruments for Special Diagnosis.... 19
II.—Generalities of Examination—General Bodily Appearance 20
III.—Observations upon Feigned, Artificially Produced, and Concealed Diseases.... 25
IV.—Rules for the Examination of Suspected Malingerers.. 30
V.—Constitutional Diseases.... 31
VI.—Diseases of Tissues.... 38
VII.—Diseases of the Cellular Tissue.... 41
VIII.—Diseases of Serous Membranes.... 42
IX.—Diseases of the Arteries.... 43
X.—Diseases of the Lymphatic System.... 43
XI.—Diseases of the Nervous System.... 44
XII.—Diseases of the Muscles, Tendons, &c.... 48
XIII.—Diseases of the Osseous System.... 49
XIV.—Pathology of Regions; Diseases of the Scalp.... 51
XV.—Diseases of the Skull.... 53
XVI.—Diseases of the Encephalon and Nervous System, Mania, Epilepsy, &c.... 54
XVII.—Diseases of the Ears.... 64
XVIII.—Diseases of the Face.... 74
XIX.—Diseases of the Eye.... 76
XX.—Diseases of the Nose and Nasal Fossæ.... 102
XXI.—Diseases of the Facial Sinus.... 106
XXII.—Diseases of the Maxillary Bones.... 106
XXIII.—Diseases of the Mouth.... 109
XXIV.—Diseases of the Neck.... 120
XXV.—Diseases of the Larynx and Trachea.... 125

SECTION		PAGE
XXVI.	—Diseases of the Pharynx	127
XXVII.	—Diseases of the Œsophagus	129
XXVIII.	—Diseases of the Cervical Vertebræ	131
XXIX.	—Diseases of the Chest and Back	132
XXX.	—Diseases of the Ribs and Sternum	136
XXXI.	—Diseases of the Clavicle and Clavicular Region	137
XXXII.	—Diseases of the Mammæ	137
XXXIII.	—Diseases of the Thoracic Organs	138
XXXIV.	—Diseases of the Spine	148
XXXV.	—Diseases of the Lumbar Region and Abdomen	153
XXXVI.	—Diseases of the Pelvis	162
XXXVII.	—Diseases of the Anus and Rectum	163
XXXVIII.	—Diseases of the Urinary Passages and Organs	168
XXXIX.	—Diseases of the Genital Organs	178
XL.	—Diseases of the Limbs	186

APPENDIX.

(OFFICIAL.)

UNITED STATES ARMY.

1. Official Instructions from the Bureau of the Provost Marshal-General for the Physical Examination of Drafted Men. 209
2. Diseases or Infirmities which Disqualify for Military Service. 211
3. Invalid Corps—Regulations for its Formation. 217
4. Invalid Corps—Physical Qualifications and Disqualifications for Admission into. 221

(OFFICIAL.)

PRUSSIAN ARMY.

5. Diseases and Disabilities causing Permanent Unfitness for Military Service. 227
6. Invalid Corps—Physical Qualifications for Admission into. 231

MANUAL OF INSTRUCTIONS

FOR

EXAMINING SURGEONS.

INTRODUCTION.

RECRUITING AS A BRANCH OF MILITARY HYGIENE.

THE profession of arms is of all others that which requires in its followers the highest degree of physical perfection. Unlike any of those connected with the civil arts, it constantly subjects the soldier to those vicissitudes of life, which are disturbing shocks to the rhythm and harmony of vital functions. From a state of passive inactivity, it suddenly calls upon him to perform long and fatiguing marches, to carry unaccustomed loads, to endure "fierce extremes" of heat, cold, and moisture, without adequate protection against their effects; to dispense with sleep when at times most exhausted, to take food at irregular and protracted intervals, and to subsist upon that which is often ill-cooked, inferior in quality, and unseasonable in character, or become unpalatable from monotony of repetition.

Yet such is the elasticity of nature in youth, that these vicissitudes, although depressing in their immediate influences, are easily recovered from, if, with a due regard to hygienic laws, the recruit is gradually broken into acquiring the habit of encountering them. While originally weak men may thus be hardened, it will always rest with commanding officers to see that due regard be had to the constitutional tendencies and the recuperative powers of their men, while inuring them to the hardships of the life they are to follow. The young may be as strong as the middle-aged, but they always differ from them in powers of endurance.

Endurance, therefore, is the result of an acquired habit of muscular activity imparting tone to the whole system. And it is the culminating point in Military Hygiene, to cultivate the physical powers of young men by a daily practice operating within the limits of their strength, and never pushing exercise beyond fatigue, nor fatigue into prostration, but pursuing its course in such a manner, as to secure a progressive development in the foundation of those powers, as well as a gradual evolution of muscular activity, so that "he who has once carried the calf may be brought to carry the ox."

No one understood this physiological law better than Napoleon, nor practised more faithfully upon it, and in illustration it is only necessary to cite the great victory of Dresden, which has been well designated a triumph of Military Hygiene.* On the afternoon of the second day of the battle, when the French army had been frequently repulsed in its attempts to cross the Elbe, the Young Guard arrived after a protracted march, beneath a sweltering heat. The moment seemed auspicious for deciding the fate of the day—the allies had long been

* Odier, Cours d'Etudes sur l'Administr. Militaire, vol. iii., p. 110. Revolat, Hygiene Militaire.

harassed by the French artillery, yet still their batteries defied the passage of the river. All eyes were now turned towards the great chief in momentary expectation of that word of command which was to dash this impetuous young host upon their obstinate foes. But the modern Cæsar understood the human constitution better than to call upon jaded troops to storm intrenchments. They were ordered to bivouac under the shade of the trees bordering the river. They were permitted to rest and refresh themselves with food and sleep until late in the day. And when at sunset they rose, a refreshed and recuperated corps, and were hurled like a thunderbolt against the enemy, the energy with which they crossed the stream, stormed the heights, and swept the Russian cannoneers from their hundred guns, testified to the wisdom of that homage which had been paid to the powers of nature. Had our generals, at the first battle of Bull Run, remembered this lesson of a great master, they too might have changed the fate of the day, and possibly shortened the life of the rebellion. How much of this wisdom of Napoleon was due to the considerate forethought of Larrey is not told us, but that he was consulted on the subject we can entertain no doubt.

In ancient no less than in modern times the selection of recruits has always been made from the most virile of the population. If a state of physical integrity be essential to the soldier at the start, that integrity must be satisfactorily ascertained beyond a peradventure, before he is admitted into the ranks. Stature and harmony of form do not alone constitute vigor of body. All modern nations understand the truth of the principle laid down by one of the earliest writers on Military Science. "*Utilius est enim fortes milites esse* *quam grandes*," and from whatever class in society taken, the recruit is always measured by his strength rather than by his size.*

It may be stated as a problem immemorially demonstrated by physiology, and deserving of consideration by economists, if only on the score of material cost, that an army recruited from the agricultural population of a country is, *cœteris paribus*, a cheaper, and at the same time more effective one than any collected from large, commercial communities. Having more physical stamina, it possesses a higher power of resistance to the causes of sickness and mortality, and presents fewer candidates for those forms of invalidism, and consequently exemption, which come from what are technically termed broken constitutions, or constitutions in which the original fund of reserved force has been exhausted—either by hereditary taints, improper education, diet, habits of occupation and life—in a word by the thousand circumstances in the midst of which civilized man lives. The ancients understood that thoroughly, and endeavored whenever possible to enforce this physical dogma. Vegetius,† writing in the

* STATURE OF THE FRENCH ARMY.

	M. C.	*Ft. I. L.*	
Infantry	1. 561	= 4 9 7½	—French measure
Riflemen	1. 761	= 5 5.	
Artillery / Engineers	1. 733	= 5 4.	
Dragoons / Lancers	1. 706	= 5 3.	
Chasseurs / Hussars	1. 679	= 5 2.	

Persons are exempt whose stature is below 1 mill. 506 cent. or 4 ft. 9 in.—ROSSIGNOL, *Traite d' Hygiene Militaire.*

† De Re Militari, lib. I., cap. iii.

time of the Emperor Valentinian, and when the influences of Asiatic conquests and the general introduction of Eastern effeminacy had enervated the Roman youth, expresses himself in the following unequivocal terms: "On which account I think no one can doubt that the rural population is best suited to bear arms, because it has been reared under the open sky and in the midst of labor. It is patient under heat—indifferent to shelter—ignorant of baths and luxuries—frugal in taste—content with little, and possesses limbs inured to every species of labor. Rural life itself accustoms men to handle implements, to dig trenches, and to bear loads. But, on the other hand, since necessity also requires that dwellers in cities should perform military duty, ere their enrolment as militia, they should be taught to run—to labor—to bear loads, and to endure heat and toil; let them also learn to live on coarse, homely fare, and to dwell now under tents, now under the sky. For I know not why it is that death is dreaded less by him who has known the least luxuries in life."

So, too, in the distribution of duties, the considerations due to age and relative strength were regarded with a scientific accuracy, and an appreciation of physiological laws which the moderns have never excelled. It would not be amiss for us to begin something similar in this respect, by distributing enlisted men among the various arms of the service according to their degree of physical vigor. Thus, instead of allowing to arbitrary and personal caprice the selection of that arm of the service in which the recruit is to enter, make it a question of physical adaptation of means to ends. Let his powers and their reach determine where he can be most useful to the country, and least exposed to fall as a sick man upon her care. Use the instruments which science has invented to disclose the latent energies that slumber out of sight, and to indicate whether his constitution foreordains him for a stout footman—a swift skirmisher—an agile horseman—a ready artificer, or a sturdy cannoneer. It is skill to be able to read his undeveloped future of power, as well as the undeveloped future of disease, which some lurking predisposition suggests. Let him be developed and improved, as well as accepted and enrolled.

SECTION I.

DUTIES OF MEDICAL EXAMINERS.

§ 1. The duties which devolve upon the examining surgeon are both delicate in their nature and of difficult performance. Intrusted with the responsibility of deciding some of the most perplexing questions in medical science upon only a few moments reflection, he cannot approach the discharge of his office without feeling how essentially important to the right understanding of every case, are the smallest apparent details of which it is made up. The causes of disease, the catenation of symptoms, their usual and ordinary progress, the results now present and visible, now unseen and latent, which they have produced in the human system—age, temperament, and occupation—all these are data which must be weighed and considered in every instance, before he can correctly form an opinion. When, in addition to the incertitude of natural phenomena, the accidents of *fraud* by simulation, or concealment, enter into the problem, it is not difficult to see that with all the skill possible, and all the readiness of observation employed, cases of deception will at times escape detection.

Instruments for Special Diagnosis.

§ 2. There are certain instruments of indispensable importance to examining surgeons, and without which none should undertake a methodical exploration of the human system. These are—

A watch (to test deafness, pulse, breathing, &c.)

Magnifying-glass (to examine the eyes and cutaneous diseases).

Spatula.

Measuring tape.

Catheter and sound.

To these may be added, for greater precision, and when time is abundant—the following, viz:

A Stethoscope.

Laryngoscope.

Speculum auris.

" ani.

Ophthalmoscope.

SECTION II.

GENERALITIES OF EXAMINATION.

§ 3. The law requiring that the recruit should be examined naked, standing, and in the day-time (*vide* Appendix), the following general rules will be found of service in beginning an examination.

General Bodily Appearance.

§ 4. The first glance at the anterior and posterior portions of the body will give the *tout ensemble*, or aggregate appearance of its conformation, and serve to answer the first interrogatory of, *faulty*, or not? The general constitutional vices, or anatomical deformities to be looked for as causes of disqualification are, *marasmus*, *obesity*, *extensive deformities of the face*, *large*, *livid*, *hairy spots*, extensive loss of substance of the *cheeks*, loss of one or both eyes—*of the nose*—of the whole or a portion of a limb—of the *testicles*, deformities of limbs, club-foot, bandy-legs, knock-knees, &c.*

§ 5. Inasmuch, however, as a simple glance is not always sufficient, a more particular and minute examination must be made, in order that whatever may have escaped the *sight*, may be discovered by the *touch*, a sense whose assistance is of infinite service in the diagnosis of many external affections.

The surgeon will therefore begin a systematic and successive examination of the various portions of the body, from the *head* downward, proceeding in each region from the exterior to the interior. Each organ should be specially interrogated by every known means, in order to ascertain—

A. If any thing interferes with that freedom and activity of its functions necessary for the performance of military duty.

B. Whether any portion of the body is incapacitated from enduring the burthen of clothing, arms, or equipments.

C. Whether from inherent debility, morbid predisposition, or existing disease, the health, and even the life

* The following description of the "good points" which the recruit should present anatomically, is so terse, comprehensive, and scientifically accurate, and stated with such elegance, and pregnant brevity, that I would not mutilate it by attempting an English paraphrase:

"Sit ergo adolescens martio operi deputandus, *vigilantibus oculis, erecta cervice, lato pectore, humeris musculosis, valentibus brachiis, digitis longioribus, ventre modicus, exilior cruribus, suris ac pedibus non superflua carne distentis, sed nervorum duritia collectis.* Cum hæc in *tyrone* signa deprehenderis, proceritatem, non magnopere desideris. Utilius est enim fortes milites esse quam grandes.—VEGETIUS, *De Re Militari*, lib. I., cap. vi.

of the individual would be endangered by the circumstances attendant upon the duties of a soldier.

D. Whether the party is suffering from any infirmity which, while not sensibly impairing organic functions, is yet so disgusting in character as to render him repulsive and uncompanionable.

§ 6. **Head.** Examine this closely for deformities, loss of substance of bones, extensive cicatrices, and cutaneous diseases. Pass the hand through the hair and ascertain whether the scalp be hot, and humid, or dry.

§ 7. **Neck.** Fulness in the region of the splenii muscles, is generally an indication of strength of body.

§ 8. **Thorax.** The thorax, particularly in its upper (clavicular and subclavian) portions affords a better index of the constitutional vigor of the individual than any other part of the body. When there is fulness, hardness, and symmetrical development of these regions and base of the neck, a presumption of constitutional soundness can safely be indulged.* On the other hand,

* Mere lack of symmetry between the sides of the chest, is not, in itself, an indication of structural change in internal organs (*e. g.*, hypertrophy, phthisis, &c.), but may be due to a variety of causes occasioning flatness of the pectoral muscles. Constantly using the right arm, or sleeping on that side, by depressing the shoulder, may give rise to this defect of uniformity.

Dr. Wm. H. Thompson, of New York, one of the State Medical Inspectors of Recruits, in his Report to the Surgeon-General, states, that "taking the whole of 5,000 observations, the *right* side was flatter than the left in 75 per cent. nearly; and out of the more marked cases of 2,000, the right side was flat in 87 per cent. . . . In 16.05 per cent., however, the left side was the flattest, though the persons were right-handed." —*Annual Report of the Surgeon-General of the State of New York*, transmitted to the Legislature, January 27th, 1863, p. 60.

Vid Woillez, Recherches pratiques sur l'Inspection et la Mensuration de la Poitrine.

sinking or depression of these parts, particularly on the left side, should always suggest the necessity of auscultation, as it is well known that the left lung suffers more commonly than the right, and that the apices and posterior parts of the upper lobes of the lungs are points of election for tubercular deposit.

Having noted these things, now measure the circumference of the chest, in its ordinary condition of intermediate expansion, by passing the tape around on a line with the nipples. This measurement should not fall below thirty-one and a half inches, nor be less than one-half of the stature of the individual. The expansive *mobility* of the chest should be from two to three inches.

The following table will explain this at a glance:

MINIMUM CIRCUMFERENCE OF THORAX TOLERABLE IN RECRUITS.*

HEIGHT. Feet.	Inches.	CIRCUMFERENCE OF THORAX. Inches.
5	3	31½
5	4	32
5	5	32½
5	6	33
5	7	33½
5	8	34
5	9	34½
5	10	35
5	11	35½
6	00	36
6	1	36½
6	2	37
6	3	37½
6	4	38

§ 9. **Abdomen.** In health the abdomen is soft, slightly convex, and its walls elastic. The regions to be examined by palpation are the right hypochondriac and epigastric, for diseases of the liver usually manifested by enlargement; left hypochondriac, for enlargement of

* *Military Hygiene*, by Brigadier-General W. A. Hammond, Surgeon-General United States Army, p. 38.

spleen, manifested by tumor and projection of the lower left ribs. Mesenteric disease reveals itself through general enlargement; while fæculent accumulations, most common in the large intestines, are shown by rough prominences in both the iliac regions.

§ 10. **Limbs.** The limbs should be free from all deformities in size, form, or relative proportion, *e. g.*, *atrophy*, *rickets*, *bandy-legs*, *knock-knees*, or *differences in length.*

§ 11. **Feet.** The feet should be arched, without deformity, or loss of substance of any of the toes, particularly the great ones.

§ 12. **Stature* and Weight.** The stature should not fall below five feet, three inches, nor the weight below that marked as its minimum accompaniment in the subjoined table:

HEIGHT. Feet.	Inches.	MINIMUM WEIGHT. lbs.
5	3	115
5	4	120
5	5	125
5	6	130
5	7	135
5	8	140
5	9	145
5	10	150
5	11	155
6	00	160
6	1	165
6	2	170
6	3	175
6	4	180
6	5	185
6	6	190
6	7	195

* Wherever there is suspicion of an attempt to decrease stature by curving the spine, the recruit should be measured supine.

SECTION III.

GENERAL OBSERVATIONS UPON FEIGNED, ARTIFICIALLY PRODUCED, AND CONCEALED DISEASES. *

§ 13. By the term *feigned disease*, is to be understood a train of symptoms provoked by artificial means, for the purpose of simulating a real disease.

An *artificially* or *self-provoked* disease exists in fact, but it is the result of criminal manœuvres performed upon the person, to avoid the discharge of some duty.

A dissembled or concealed disease, is one which, although existing in fact, is purposely concealed with an intention to defraud observation.

The military surgeon should always be on his guard against *feigned* diseases, as well among soldiers seeking for a discharge, as among recruits; and also be vigilant to detect *dissembled* or concealed diseases in substitutes and volunteers.

* For exhaustive details on this subject, the surgeon will do well to consult, ZACCHIAS, Quæstiones Medico-Legales, lib. III., tit. II.; FODERE, Medecine-Légale, vol. 2, p. 457; MAHON, Medecine-Légale, vol. 1, p. 324; DEVERGIE, Medecine-Légale, vol. 1, p. 605; BECK'S Medical Jurisprudence, vol. 1, art. "Feigned Diseases;" CASPER, Medecine-Légale, vol. 1, p. 238; PERCY and LAURENT in Dict. des Sciences-Médicales, art. "Simulation;" Cyclopædia of Practical Medicine, art. "Feigned Diseases;" COPLAND'S Dictionary of Practical Medicine, art. "Feigning Disease;" DUNGLISON'S Medical Dictionary, art. "Feigned Disease."

Artificially Produced Diseases.

§ 14. Artificially produced diseases which, as we have seen, are diseases in fact, occasion the greatest perplexity to the surgeon, by reason of their rarely disclosing the sources of their origin; and in general it is only when recent, that their origin can at all be discovered. In doubtful cases the surgeon will have to resort to all the questions enumerated below. (§ 23.)

Dissembled, or Concealed Diseases.

§ 15. The duty of the surgeon in exploring a party to discover dissembled or concealed diseases, is always a difficult one, for many diseases having their seat in internal organs, when they have not produced constitutional, nor sympathetic disturbances, will often escape observation. This is particularly the case with intermittent affections, which may exist undiscovered so long as the surgeon does not himself witness a paroxysm.

Feigned Diseases.

§ 16. In treating of simulation in connection with the various diseases which are hereafter to be enumerated, the methods of *detecting* fraud will alone be given.* It cannot be necessary to a surgeon experienced in the physiognomy of disease to be told what and how many are

* As these pages cannot be restricted in their circulation to the hands of surgeons alone, it has been deemed judicious to exclude from them all enumeration of the *pharmacopœia* and the *enginery* from which simulators draw their means of deception. The sources of information touching these practices are well known to all physicians, and elsewhere pointed out, and aside from policy, it would only augment the size of this manual without adding to its usefulness to enter into the pathogeny of feigned diseases.

the particular agencies which criminal design employs to impose upon his credulity. The differential diagnosis of the real and the feigned disease will rarely fail to expose the incongruity existing between the actual and the alleged malady. The ignorance of symptomatology—of sympathetic, and consequential manifestations—of the law of periodicity—of the co-ordination of vital forces and functions—in a word, of anatomy and physiology, renders the majority of simulators mere physical clowns. The rationale of simulation being a travesty of natural phenomena and a violation of truth, in its details, generally exposes itself at a glance to the prying, skilled eye of science. Nevertheless, we must not despise the class entirely. There are some experts in it, and even physicians have been found in other countries selling their knowledge in this way, and prostituting their skill to the basest of purposes, by instructing malingerers in the use of harmful drugs, and in the performance of criminal manipulations, calculated to impair, temporarily, their vigor of body. But in all cases the surgeon must be prepared to meet the simulator on his own ground, and if need be, *superare malitiam malitia*, by artfully circumventing him.

§ 17. For obvious reasons, chronic forms of disease are of preference feigned by malingerers. As it is known among recruits that the examination of the surgeon must, of necessity, be brief—that it cannot be repeated, but must terminate his inquiry once for all, it is naturally supposed that the more numerous the symptoms they can present the greater will be the bias of a first impression in favor of their disability. Others select milder forms of diseases whenever they mistrust their ability to simulate their acute type, alleging with much reiteration, that they have been worse even than they now are, and that the surgeon sees their malady under its most favorable aspect. This is commonly the case when *rheumatism*, *neuralgic pains*, *chronic piles*, *lumbago*, *diseases of the bladder or kidneys*, *constant severe headache*, *ulcers*, *deafness*, *old sprains*, &c., &c., are feigned.

§ 18. The following synoptical table exhibits feigned diseases under three pathogenetic classifications, viz.:

A. Such as depend upon the influence of the *will* upon muscles of voluntary motion.

B. Such as are excited by artificial agents without lesion of tissues.

C. Such as are similarly excited with lesion of tissues.

A. Class First.

§ 19. Feigned diseases depending upon the influence of will upon muscles of voluntary motion, and an impaired state of the animal functions.

Epilepsy, idiocy, loss of memory, mania, deafness, ptosis of right eyelid, involuntary and convulsive movements of the eyes, or their lids, strabismus, dumbness, aphonia, stammering, torticollis, curvature of the spine, voluntary vomiting, rumination, retention, and incontinence of urine, general or partial tremor, paralysis, retraction, or continuous flexion of fingers and limbs, lameness, unnatural elevation of one shoulder, partial or complete anchylosis of a limb, inversion or torsion of one foot.

B. Class Second.

§ 20. Feigned diseases imitated by artificial means and presenting as yet no alteration of tissues nor important lesion of functions.

Jaundice, ecchymosis, phthiriasis, purulent discharge from ears, hæmoptysis, hæmatemesis, hæmaturia, internal piles, prolapsus ani, excretion of vesical calculi, varices, hæmorrhoidal flux.

C. Class Third.

§ 21. Feigned diseases, voluntarily excited, and imitated by the internal or external use of agents, capable of producing an unnatural change in the form, volume, integrity, continuity, and sensibility of different parts of the body.

Wounds, mutilations, ulcers, cutaneous diseases, and petechiæ, ophthalmia, scurvy of gums, caries, partial or total loss of teeth, vertigo, mania, emphysema, ascites, tympanites, hydrocele, vomiting of food, syncope, feebleness of pulse, palpitation of heart, amaurosis, fever, emaciation.

Diseases which may be Concealed.

§ 22. Incontinence of fæces, rheumatism and neuralgic pains, prolapsus ani, retention or incontinence of urine, shortening of an inferior extremity, loss of memory, epilepsy, somnambulism, periodical hæmoptysis, asthma, tænia, habitual vomiting, gravel or hæmorrhoidal flux, chronic catarrh of bladder, intermittent fever, syphilis.

SECTION IV.

RULES FOR THE EXAMINATION OF SUSPECTED MALINGERERS.

§ 23. Whenever a disease is alleged to exist, by a recruit, the first duty of the surgeon is to determine whether it be of such a character as admits of being *feigned*. This is the starting point of all subsequent inquiry.

A. In cases of doubt, it is always safest to assume the disease as feigned, rather than as real, and to proceed to a minute and detailed examination of the party with all possible delicacy and moderation, and without any seeming suspicion.

B. If the history and symptoms of the alleged disease, and the changes wrought by it in the economy, are at variance with the regular and ordinary course of the true disease, simulation may be suspected.

C. The party should be questioned in relation to symptoms, in order to test their correspondence with those usually present in similar diseases, and by leading him on vaguely, with irrelevant inquiries touching other disorders, he will often, if a malingerer, expose himself by confounding symptoms belonging to dissimilar and opposite diseases.

D. In investigating an internal malady, assume to believe in the existence of all the symptoms narrated; then apply the rule *contraria contrariis*, and ask leading and suggestive questions touching the presence of incongruous symptoms, such as amblyopia, hæmorrhage from the left ear, swelling of the thumbs (Casper), coldness of the tongue, &c. The simulator will often entrap himself by an affirmative reply, based upon the supposition that he had mis-stated the symptoms of his malady and can now correct his mistake by adopting new ones.*

E. By calling attention away from himself, the party may often be made to perform acts entirely incompatible with the existence of his alleged disease, and thus expose his deception.

SECTION V.

CONSTITUTIONAL DISEASES.

§ 24. Whatever may have been said in favor of, or against temperaments, and whatever the disputes in relation to their classification, it is an admitted fact, that in every age, and among all men, they have been recognized as influencing the predisposition to disease.† On this account, therefore, if no other, the surgeon should interrogate them as sources of æteological influence. For, the physical aspect presented by the body in this particular expresses the predominance or exaggeration of either the *sanguineous*, *lymphatic*, or *nervous* systems, and the consequent predisposition to those diseases

* Ut ergo prudens Medicus ad decernendum ab ipsis Jurisconsultis de veritate vocatus, non decipiatur, plura in consideratione adhibeat necesse est; et primo partem quæ dolet, vel quæ dolore simulatur; secundò doloris speciem; tertio causam doloris, et maximè siquam enarravit patiens ex procatarcticis et externis; quarto doloris ipsius durationem; quinto remedia adhibita seu adhibenda.—*Zacchias*, Op. cit., lib. III., tit. II., q. IV.

† Military Hygiene, by Brigadier-General Wm. A. Hammond, Surgeon General U. S. A., page 78.

having their origin in one of these three great centres. Hence, in the lymphatic, we look for diseases of the glandular system; in the sanguine, for diseases of the circulation; and, in the nervous, for diseases reflected from preternatural irritability of the cerebro-spinal system upon large organs, like the stomach, brain, or heart. But, inasmuch as there are no pure or unmixed temperaments, no absolute deductions can be drawn from the foregoing classes, though in each case, taking temperament only as a relative element in the computation, we shall still find it acting as an important postulate to predisposition.

Sources of Indication.

§ 25. There are three sources through which radical constitutional impairment ever exhibits itself externally, viz.:

1st. Through the *glandular* system, producing the true strumous diathesis.

2d. Through the *osseous* system, giving rise to rickets and rickety deformities.

3d. Through the *skin*, giving rise to obstinate cutaneous diseases.

Whenever these manifestations have plainly existed to such a degree and for such a length of time as to indicate a chronic impairment of the functions of nutrition and secretion, it is evident that such a state borders on actual disease, and unfits the party for military service.

Feebleness of Constitution.

§ 26. Without the existence of special disease in any organ or tissue of the body, there may yet be presented by an examination of the person, such proofs of a *want of tone* and of *powers of endurance*, and such an absence of *recuperative force and of vigor in vital functions*, as to show that the constitution could not rally against causes of depression, nor promptly re-establish itself with the spontaneity due to plenitude of original vigor. This condition, popularly designated as feebleness of constitution, cannot always be defined with precision, because in each individual, the circumstances of *absolute* and *reserved vigor* express themselves through different physical phenomena, and what might be relative weakness in one, born of habits of life, and occupation, temporary and remediable, would in another indicate congenital absence of tone. It is idle to suppose that constitutions can be re-cast. Original nature may be modified, but never entirely altered. We must judge of the vigor of the human edifice by the character of its foundation, for where this is weak, the superstructure, however beautiful, is only calculated to deceive us. The following are manifestations which generally accompany feebleness of constitution: *Excessive stature without corresponding breadth of person; long, thin neck*; *narrow chest*, *sunken* or *flattened; shrunken abdomen; flaccidity*, *without development of the belly of large muscles; limbs larger at the joints than in the centre*, *articulations coarse; skin soft and flabby*, *and almost barren of hair; lips pale*, and a general indication of want of activity in the vital functions.

Although many of these conditions are presented during convalescence from acute affections, yet the skilful surgeon will readily detect, by the degree to which the constitution is affected, whether the diathesis presented by the party be *radical* or merely *accidental* in its character.

Anæmia.

§ 27. Anæmia, characterized by general debility, emaciation, flaccidity, and pallor of tissues, sometimes even infiltration of the cellular tissue and souffle in the carotids, can only justify the rejection of a recruit when it is of the gravest character. Misery, certain professions followed in dark and damp places, labor disproportioned to strength, venereal excesses, scurvy, convalescence from acute diseases, are all determining causes of this diathesis, which is removable under proper hygienic and therapeutic treatment. Rejection in such case must rest upon the question of extent of disease, and probable time required to recover from it. Anæmia may be artificially produced, but not feigned.

Scrofula.

§ 28. Scrofula, when unmodified by the influences of puberty, and characterized by glandular enlargements, or ulcerations in the *cervical* or *submaxillary* regions, is a disease of sufficient gravity to justify rejection. When, however, this diathesis, united to an otherwise tolerable state of health, is little developed and constitutes more of a predisposition than a positive disease, and in particular when this predisposition seems to arise rather from the bad hygienic conditions in the midst of which the party has lived, it often happens that the change of habitation, diet, and occupation, essentially improve the waning constitution, and convert into a healthy soldier a civilian, whose mode of life otherwise doomed him to the infirmities born of scrofula.

This constitutional vice is indicated by slight puffiness of the face, thin, transparent skin, through which the veins appear prominent, *the alæ nasi are smooth and tumefied, the upper lip thickened, the limbs are rounded, the flesh soft and flaccid, and the abdomen slightly enlarged.* In a more advanced stage, the *eyelids are swollen, red, everted* (blear-eyed) *with discharge from the meibomian glands*, and the ears surrounded by suppurative crusts.

Although malingerers sometimes attempt to simulate scrofula, by making irritating applications to the eyelids, nose, and upper lip, the absence of all constitutional complications readily exposes the cheat. Besides which scrofulous ulcers and scars have a specific character, the former having pale and flabby borders, with thin edges, and discharging a serous matter, mixed with grumous, cheesy clots; and the latter being deep, adherent to the subcutaneous tissue, bluish colored when recent; white when old, irregular with transverse bridles, and being found in the track of the lymphatic ganglions. The same degree of scrofula which justifies rejection, likewise justifies discharge.

Syphilis.

§ 29. Primary or local syphilis does not justify rejection, unless accompanied by extensive ulcers, calculated to leave large, feeble, irregular cicatrices, and much loss of substance. The same is not the case with secondary syphilis, which denotes a true venereal saturation of the constitution, and is marked by profound alteration of the vital functions, engorgement of the cervical, axillary, inguinal, and lymphatic ganglions, ulcerations of the mucous membrane of the nose, caries of the bones, &c., in those whose constitutions are seriously affected by it. This condition of body, although curable under skilful treatment, yet indicates such impairment of the constitution, as renders it certain that the party cannot withstand the duties and hardships of a military life. He must be rejected.

Scurvy.

§ 30. Scurvy, which is never congenital, but always acquired, presents itself under different degrees of intensity. The judgment of the surgeon will accordingly be guided by the peculiar phases it reveals, in determining the questions of rejection or discharge. In slight cases, and where the morbid manifestations are simply local, improved hygienic conditions will usually suffice to produce a rapid recovery. But when the disease has assumed a serious form, and is accompanied by fungous gums, falling of the teeth, œdema of the limbs, discoloration of the tissues, serous infiltration, petechiæ, passive hæmorrhage, and muscular pains, the recruit must be rejected.

Cachexies.

§ 31. Various cachexies resulting from malarious, lead, or mercurial poisoning, or others arising from the practice of certain avocations, may also come under the notice of the surgeon. So long as there is no manifest impairment of the constitution, and a change of habits and occupation seems likely to insure a recovery, rejection is unjustifiable. But when alterations in structure have resulted, or organic functions are so unsettled as to fall readily into morbid conditions under slight exciting causes, the recruit must be rejected. The same rule will apply to discharges.

These cachexies may be artificially produced, but cannot be feigned.

Tuberculosis.

§ 32. Tubercles, although most commonly exhibiting themselves in the lungs, or peritoneum, are yet often found in other tissues. Their deposition depends upon a peculiar diathesis, which manifestly impairs the constitutional vigor necessary for the military service. In their second stage (that of softening and suppuration) their diagnosis is easy. But in their first stage, where they remain in the form of a hard, indolent, isolated deposit, producing no sensible disturbance of any of the organic functions, they may escape observation. It is different with masses of tubercles which even in their first stage are generally appreciable. It is through the constitutional manifestations that the sur geon must seek for revelations of this diathesis where-ever he suspects its existence.

Melanosis.

§ 33. Melanosis which is a deposit of black pigment in the tissue of diseased organs, does not differ greatly from cancer, and when occurring in encephaloid structures, constitutes true melanoid cancer. At times it occurs in organs not essentially diseased.

Any attempt at feigning this affection by introducing coloring pigments beneath the skin, is of so gross a nature as to readily expose itself.

Cancer.

§ 34. Several morbid conditions of structure essentially different in their anatomical elements, are confounded under the common designation of cancer—such, for example, as *scirrhus*, *encephaloid*, *and colloid cancer*. Whatever its seat or nature, cancer ever presents itself under the form of a fungous growth, tumor, or of open ulcerations. Being always a serious affection, with disposition to recurrence when locally extirpated, its diagnosis becomes of the greatest importance to the surgeon, and as this is at times extremely difficult, all his sagacity will be required in arriving at a conclusion in the premises.

The first thing to be remembered is that cancer is of rare occurrence in youth, and, secondly, that it cannot be feigned. In recruits, therefore, the presumptions are against it; in old soldiers it is different; but in both classes rejection or discharge must follow upon its detection. The liability to alteration of the lymphatic glands in the vicinity of the suspected cancerous disease is to be borne in mind as a characteristic sign.

Cancroid and Fibro-plastic Tumors.

§ 35. The same rules which apply to cancer, will apply to cancroid and fibro-plastic tumors. These, although differing from the former in anatomical features, yet engender the like disability for military service.

SECTION VI.

DISEASES OF TISSUES.

Diseases of the Skin.—Eczema and Lichen.

§ 36. If slight and acute, neither of these affections are necessarily disqualifications for military service, but when become chronic and extensive, the recruit must be rejected, and the soldier discharged.

All chronic and extensive diseases of the skin of parasitic origin, are causes of rejection, because of their contagiousness, unless the circumstances of the service require that the recruit should be accepted and sent to the hospital for cure.

Erysipelas.

§ 37. This affection, whenever it has produced serious results, may require the rejection of the recruit. Ordinarily it does not.

Artificially Produced Exanthemata.

§ 38. Certain articles of food, varieties of shell-fish in particular, may be used to provoke eruptions and to deceive the surgeon. It is only necessary to allude to this as a possibility not to be overlooked.

Ulcers.

§ 39. Although ulcers generally exhibit themselves upon the inferior extremities, and are there also oftenest feigned or artificially produced, they may, whatever their nature, appear upon other parts of the body. They justify rejection only when their chronic character is well established, and they co-exist with a morbid diathesis. Artificially produced ulcers eventually assume the character of chronic ones, and may, by the lesions they have produced, in like manner justify rejection, for at this stage of their existence it is impossible to distinguish them from spontaneous ones. When factitious ulcers have not deeply altered the surrounding tissues, they can readily be discovered by the following features.

In old ulcers the epidermis is shiny, hairless, and of a violet color, this latter fading by insensible gradations into that of the healthy skin. In recent artificially produced ulcers, the wound is circumscribed, and marked by a distinct circle. Where the party appears in good health, and without emaciation—where the cervical lymphatic ganglions are not enlarged, and where the edges of the ulcer are round and brown, the base red and purplish, and the surrounding tissue inflamed, spotted, or exhibiting blisters, there is presumption of criminal agency in their production, for men suffering from old ulcers are generally cachectic, having the skin dry and scaly; and where the sore has attacked a limb, this often becomes atrophied or œdematous.

Nævi Materni, Erectile Tumors.

§ 40. The former can only justify rejection when sufficiently large to constitute, especially on the face, disgusting hideousness. The latter consisting of vascular tissue, formed in the capillary system of the chorion, and often on the surface of mucous membranes in the vicinity of natural openings, may justify rejection, if extensive, and situated on such parts of the body as are exposed to blows or habitual pressure.

Cicatrices.

§ 41. All extensive, irregular, unyielding cicatrices, causing notable changes in the relations of parts, uniting contiguous organs, and interfering with freedom of muscular exercise, justify both rejection and discharge.

Steatomatous Tumors.

§ 42. Moles, warts, or wens of large growth, likewise

justify rejection when present in a region exposed to pressure, and when they interfere with freedom of motion in adjacent parts.

SECTION VII.

DISEASES OF THE CELLULAR TISSUE.

Leanness and Emaciation.

§ 43. Leanness, by itself, is not a cause for rejection, when present in an otherwise sound constitution. But when it attains to the degree of emaciation, and borders on marasmus, it must be considered as a disqualification for military service.

Obesity.

§ 44. Obesity as a general thing justifies rejection, but a mere predisposition to it does not, on the presumption that an active life would interfere with its further development.

Anasarca and Œdema.

§ 45. The former of these conditions is ordinarily symptomatic of visceral disease, and as such requires that the recruit be rejected. When, however, the affection is acute and primitive, no opinion should be hastily pronounced; the party being meanwhile provisionally remanded until time shall decide the question.

Œdema being a local infiltration of the cellular tissue likewise dependent on visceral disease, derives all its importance from the character of the organ primarily affected. When primitive in its nature, and arising from merely accidental causes, as for example sudden cold, it is without importance. The source of its origin must determine the question of disability.

Abscesses.

§ 46. **Acute Abscesses** justify rejection only when extensive, producing exhaustion, suppuration, and great loss of substance.

Chronic Idiopathic Abscesses, the indicia of a confirmed scrofulous diathesis, always justify rejection.

Cold Abscesses, being always symptomatic of grave lesions in deep seated parts, are absolute causes for rejection.

Fatty and Encysted Tumors.

§ 47. The size, extent, and position of these formations, with relation to the pressure likely to be made upon them by clothing and equipments, must determine the question of rejection.

SECTION VIII.

DISEASES OF SEROUS MEMBRANES.

Dropsy.

§ 48. Dropsy, situated in any of the splanchnic cavities, always requires that the recruit be rejected. Discharges are to be granted only after treatment has proved unavailing.

SECTION IX.

DISEASES OF THE ARTERIES.

Aneurism.

§ 49. Aneurisms, which are tumors formed by arterial blood, consist either in a dilatation of the walls of an artery without rupture (*true aneurism*), or dilatation with rupture and escape of blood into adjacent tissues (*false or diffused*, *circumscribed aneurism*), or passage of the blood from an open artery into a vein (aneurismal varix). Either of these conditions is a cause for rejection. When declaring itself in soldiers, it is equally a cause for discharge.

SECTION X.

DISEASES OF THE LYMPHATIC SYSTEM.

§ 50. Dilatation of the lymphatic vessels is occasionally met with, and requires rejection whenever it is extensive.

Angeioloceutis.

§ 51. Inflammation of the lymphatic vessels is not a serious affection in its acute stage, and is not a disqualification for military service. In its chronic stage it is extremely rare, and its symptoms obscure, yet when discovered to exist, is a cause for rejection.

Lymphatic Adenitis.

§ 52. Acute adenitis, usually running its course in a

few days, is not in general a cause for rejection. If, however, it be considerable, it may produce extensive detachment of parts, fistulas, &c., requiring a long period for recovery, and consequently disables the party for military service. In each case the judgment of the surgeon must be exercised in arriving at a conclusion. Chronic adenitis is often evidence of constitutional disease in itself justifying rejection.

SECTION XI.

DISEASES OF THE NERVOUS SYSTEM.

Paralysis.

§ 53. This affection, which is easily feigned, may be restricted to one limb, to a few muscles, or it may extend over a large portion of the body, as in *hemiplegia* and *paraplegia*.

When it involves any considerable portion of the muscular system, there is always to be noticed flaccidity and flabbiness of the flesh, with, often, a beginning of atrophy, discoloration of the skin, weakness of the articulations, and more or less alteration of the sensibility. The normal temperature is ordinarily lowered in a paralyzed part, and the general physiognomy of paralysis is such that it cannot be counterfeited, so as to deceive a practised eye. This is particularly the case in hemiplegia and paraplegia, affections referable for their origin to the brain and spinal marrow. In cases of suspected feigning, the truth may be discovered by employing either surprises or painful applications borrowed from the class of remedial agents proper to the treatment of real paralysis, as for example the cold douche.

In making a diagnosis, it is necessary to distinguish between paralysis of the nerves of sensation and those of motion. Unexpected wounding of the former will readily expose deception, and paralyses of central origin are accompanied by general symptoms which cannot be imitated. It is otherwise with feigned paralysis of the motor nerves, which is extremely difficult to detect. The keenest observation and scrutiny will here be required.

Lead Paralysis.

§ 54. Under the influence of emanations from lead, and consequently in those professions in which this metal is used, artisans are exposed to a form of paralysis which exhibits itself in different muscles of the trunk and extremities, with this characteristic feature, viz.: that only a certain number of muscles are affected. Although the paralysis may be incomplete, as regards the whole limb, it is always complete as regards the muscles involved in it. The extensors are those which most generally suffer. The limbs remain in a semi-flexed position (as for example, the hand upon the fore-arm), the patient not being able to extend them without assistance from another limb, or by pressure against some solid body. Inquiries into the vocation of the individual, and particularly as to whether he had ever suffered an attack of lead-colic, a symptom nearly always preceding this form of paralysis, will serve greatly to illumine the judgment of the surgeon. Besides which, the peculiar diathesis which accompanies such cases—the blue line on the edge of the gums, spots on the mucous membrane, with occasional amaurotic complications, and the visible impairment in the function of nutrition, leave little room for doubt. Rejection follows of necessity.

Paralysis from Fatty Degeneration.

§ 55. Paralysis may result from fatty degeneration of the muscles, producing insensibility to the influences of the nervous fluid, and deformity, or deviation of the limbs.

Traumatic Paralysis.

§ 56. The diagnosis of this form of paralysis is extremely difficult. In such cases, the parts must be critically explored for scars or deformities, and to discover whether any important nerve has been wounded, and thus afford some anatomical reason for the paralysis. The patient must also be questioned in relation to the connection between these two circumstances. It must not be forgotten that traumatic paralysis, as well as that arising from internal or spontaneous causes, gives rise, when prolonged, to marked changes in the nutrition of the affected parts, and that the absence of these indicia creates a just suspicion of simulation.

General Progressive Paralysis.

§ 57. General progressive paralysis manifests itself through enfeeblement of the muscular system, increasing difficulty of articulation, tremor of the limbs, and atrophy of the muscles. These phenomena, originally insidious in their inception, progress steadily until at a later stage the muscles of organic life participate in the general paralysis. This condition, which cannot be feigned, necessitates rejection.

Habitual Tremor.

§ 58. Emanations from lead as well as mercury, producing a real lead or mercurial poisoning in those constantly exposed to them, frequently give rise to *partial* or *general* tremor. This constitutional condition, denoting, as it does, lesion in some of the nervous centres, always disqualifies its subjects for military service. It is rare that this state can be feigned with any success, because of the characteristic features of the affection. The muscular spasms which it occasions are short, irregular, in a word, clonic; any attempt at flexion of a limb being preceded by short snatches of unsuccessful effort, occasioning tremor and involuntary agitation. Wherever there is suspicion of simulation, close questioning must be resorted to.

Partial Atrophy.

§ 59. The same rule as to rejection, applies to partial atrophy of the muscular system, with or without fatty degeneration, unless the atrophy, united to unimpaired constitutional vigor, is inextensive and confined to muscles of secondary importance.

Permanent Contractions.

§ 60. Permanent contractions, rigidity, and shortening of certain muscles, with diminution or loss of their normal extensibility, occasions sometimes flexion, and more rarely permanent extension of a limb. Such states are always disqualification for military service. Contractions of the neck, spinal column, and limbs, are often feigned, which facts reveal themselves whenever, although alleged to be of ancient date, no emaciation of the involved tissues presents itself. *Essential contrac-*

tion, better known as *intermittent tetanus*, is of such difficult diagnosis as often to escape observation; the short time allowed the surgeon for examination not affording sufficient opportunity for the complete study of a disease but recently known. It is always a cause for rejection or discharge.

Neuroma.

§ 61. These painful pisiform tumors, seated in the subcutaneous nervous twigs, are always a cause for rejection when they can be detected externally.

SECTION XII.

DISEASES OF MUSCLES, TENDONS AND THEIR SHEATHS.

Rupture of Muscles, (coup de fouet).

§ 62. Simple rupture of muscular fibres is generally inconsequential in its results, and affords no cause for rejection.

Retraction and Rupture of Tendons.

§ 63. *Retractions and ruptures* of tendons modify the anatomical relations of the muscles to which they are attached, exercise an energetic action upon the direction of bones, and produce more or less obstacle to the freedom of motion. In such cases exemption must be granted.

Affections of Tendinous Ganglia.

§ 64. Inflammation and dropsy of tendinous ganglia,

vary in gravity according to their extent and seat. The surgeon will determine whether or not they entitle to rejection by their degree, and the changes they have wrought in parts.

SECTION XIII.

OSSEOUS SYSTEM.

Diseases of Bones and their Articulations.

§ 65. The bones are subject to many forms of lesion and alteration, which may be briefly enumerated as follows, viz:

1st. Such as are incurable.

2d. Such as, though variable in character and more or less curable, are, like the former, causes of absolute disability for military service.

3d. Such as furnish only probable causes for either rejection or discharge.

Incurable Affections.

§ 66. Foremost among these may be enumerated *rachitic curvatures*, *alterations* in shape or *shortening* of the long bones, *spina ventosa*, *osteo-sarcoma*, *false articulations* arising from un-united fractures or ill-reduced luxations, articular distentions arising from violent sprains, luxations or relaxations of capsular ligaments, and complete or partial *anchylosis* of important articulations.

In this connection it is well to remark that partial anchylosis is often feigned. When real, the *shape* of the joint most generally reveals traces of the inflammation, wounds, or fractures it has suffered, phenomena not observable in simulated cases. In true anchylosis, motion which is free within the limits described by the lesion, ceases suddenly when beyond them, as though met by an inert, hard obstacle, and without any intervention of muscular opposition. Auscultation during motion often detects a characteristic shock when the limit is reached. Motion is not painful, nor does its extent ever vary Malingerers generally complain of pain on motion. They stiffen the limb, arrest its motion at different angles, and by contraction of its muscles, easily perceived through their hardness and the tense state of their tendons, disclose the simulation they are practising.

INFIRMITIES OF THE SECOND CLASS.

Necrosis and Caries.

§ 67. *Necrosis* and *caries*, *fistulas* arising from bony cavities, the substance of bones, or from articulations; *chronic enlargements*, *white swellings*, hydarthrosis, and *floating cartilages* in joints.

INFIRMITIES OF THE THIRD CLASS.

Periostosis and Exostosis..

§ 68. Neither of these affections, whether of idiopathic or traumatic origin, necessarily justify rejection, unless they are so situated as to be painfully compressed during decubitus, or to hinder the motion of parts. When dependent upon syphilis they usually occupy by preference certain localities which readily distinguish them from those of different origin.

SECTION XIV.

PATHOLOGY OF REGIONS.

Diseases of the Scalp—Tinea Capitis and its Varieties.

§ 69. These diseases being all more or less related to a cachectic habit of body, must be considered as so many exponents of an impaired constitution. They will justify rejection or discharge whenever it is manifest from their gravity, that the source of their origin is incurably contaminated, as well as on account of their contagiousness. Chronic *tinea*, *favosa*, and *scutulata*, always justify rejection or discharge. Tinea *furfuracea*, when slight, does not.

Eczema and Impetigo.

§ 70. These diseases are often feigned by the application of irritants to the scalp. But the fraud is easily detected in such cases, since the characteristic odor of the disease is wanting, the crusts are not depressed, and when detached, a healthy circumscribed wound with an inflammatory areola is seen, the other portions of the scalp being sound.

When these diseases are attempted to be concealed, they may still be detected, after thoroughly cleansing the head, by the hot, humid feeling of the scalp; and if the hair be separated, erosions more or less deep, and other indicia of vesicular inflammation, will be discovered. Examination of the scalp by the eye and touch should never be omitted.

Baldness.

§ 71. Extensive baldness requires, on many accounts,

that the recruit should be rejected. Whenever this takes place naturally, the denuded surface is smooth, shining, and of a white or yellowish tinge. The utmost scrutiny fails to detect the bluish points corresponding to the openings of the hair-bulbs. Sometimes superficial cicatrices of various size resulting from the effects of *favus* may be noted. Whenever artificial means have been employed to produce baldness, however carefully the operation may have been performed, the tegument of the scalp will never wear the appearance described above. Its surface, on the contrary, has a dull, unvarnished look, like the rest of the skin, and on a critical examination, the openings of the hair-bulbs are plainly discernible.

Passing the hand over the head, will never fail to detect the existence of artificial appliances, if any are attached to the surface of the scalp.

Tumors.

§ 72. *Wens*, *erectile*, *fibrous*, and *fungous* tumors, scrofulous abscesses, abscesses by congestion, are all causes for rejection on account of the impediment they present to, or the pain which they cause in wearing the military head-dress. The same rule will not apply to *acute* abscesses, unless they are of great size; nor to tumors resulting from simple contusions, and curable in a few days.

Cicatrices.

§ 73. Extensive, irregular, and slightly consolidated cicatrices, occupying a large surface of the scalp, may, for the reasons given above, justify rejection.

SECTION XV.

DISEASES OF THE SKULL.

Want of Development and Malconformation.

§ 74. Size being generally a measure of power, an exceedingly small or deformed skull, limiting the mass of the brain, becomes, inferentially, an index of feeble intelligence. The apparent *volume* of the brain, rather than the *shape* of the skull, should guide the surgeon in this matter, which, after all, becomes important only when there is marked vicious conformation of the latter.

Incomplete Ossification.

§ 75. Incomplete ossification of the skull is revealed through the persistence of the fronto-parietal fontanelle, or sometimes by the non-union, mobility, and elastic depressibility of the edges of the bones. It is always a disqualification for the military service.

Fractures and Loss of Substance.

§ 76. Old fractures, although perfectly healed, when they leave any predisposition to disease, are absolute causes for rejection.

Loss of substance of any of the bones, arising either from wounds, trephining, caries, or necrosis, is also a disqualification for military service.

Tumors.

§ 77. Certain fungous tumors, having their origin in the bones of the skull, and appearing prominently beneath the scalp, are generally causes for rejection, unless they are so small and benign in character as to provoke no inconvenience. But when these tumors are evidently seated beneath the external table, they are absolute disqualifications for military service.

SECTION XVI.

DISEASES OF THE ENCEPHALON AND NERVOUS SYSTEM.

§ 78. The difficulty of discovering many anomalous conditions of the brain, which are just causes of disqualification in a recruit, and yet are unrevealed, except through the instrumentality of organs largely controlled by the will, renders this department of observation one in which *feigning* can be undertaken with many chances of success. Although public report generally stigmatizes the mentally degraded with a species of notoriety, yet the surgeon may have no means of ascertaining this, and must, therefore, resort to such physical signs as are revealed through the physiognomy, shape of the head, general demeanor, and conversation.

Idiocy.

§ 79. Idiocy, which is a congenital deficiency of mind, is generally marked by a peculiar type of expression which cannot be mistaken. This is particularly the case when the deficiency exists in the highest degree. Both this state and its minor condition, termed imbecility, are disqualifications for military service.

Mania and Dementia.

§ 80. Mania* manifests itself under a variety of forms, which it must suffice only to name in this connection. Thus *melancholia*, *monomania*, including under this latter homicidal and suicidal mania; kleptomania, erotomania, &c., &c., are all varieties of the same disorder.

Dementia, on the other hand, or as it has well been termed, "the tomb of the human reason," is the last stage of degradation into which a mind, originally developed, can fall. It is the opposite pole to idiocy, which is always congenital, while dementia is acquired.

The delicate shades of mental aberration, observed in the varieties of mania, are at times of such difficult recognition, that a most assiduous and prolonged examination, frequently repeated, is necessary to enable the physician to arrive at any opinion in the premises. In many cases the symptoms are so manifest and out-spoken as to leave no doubt of the presence or character of the disorder. But in the majority of cases, and where no adequate time is allowed for examination, the surgeon will find himself laboring under great perplexity. The only general rules of examination which can be given for such cases are these: To converse with the suspected party on general subjects, rapidly passing from one class to another, and suggesting in particular such as are mutually incompatible, and doing this in such a way as not to give time for the preparation of special answers; to seize upon any word which escapes him, and seems to have anticipated reflection, and by surprising him,

* Mania, in some of its many forms, has been the chosen disease of simulators in all ages. That royal malingerer, the crafty Ulysses, feigned it in order to avoid going to the siege of Troy. King David, Junius Brutus, and Solon also practised this deception for various purposes.

possibly secure a self-contradiction. At the same time the physiognomy, gestures, and demeanor, style of clothing and appearance are all to be studied, in order to ascertain whether they agree or disagree with the conditions of mind in which he is suspected to be. Observation made of him while engaged in conversation with others, sometimes concealing from him the object of these interviews, and sometimes again revealing it to him, will all contribute something to the data upon which the surgeon is to found his opinion.

There is, generally speaking, a marked difference between the truly insane man and the simulator, while undergoing an examination, whose character and object he is informed of. The truly insane, on such occasions, feels hurt at the imputation cast upon his sanity, and makes desperate efforts to appear well and answer correctly; while the simulator does not repel with equal force the imputation of insanity, and generally overacts the symptoms which he supposes belong to this condition of mind. The patient should unexpectedly be examined at night, and on different occasions, in order to ascertain the condition of his sleep. Yet too much stress is occasionally laid upon insomnolence, as one of the characteristic symptoms of insanity. This condition belongs more particularly to *mania*, in which disease patients always suffer from broken, feverish, and interrupted slumbers,* while in the false maniac there is true sleep, resulting from the exhaustion produced by a day of feigned agitation; and in proportion as the

* It is well to bear in mind the distinction between *sleep* and *slumber*. As a general rule, the insane never *sleep* soundly. But as a class, they all slumber more or less.

symptoms feigned have been tumultuous and exhaustive, will the sleep be profound.

In *dementia*, on the contrary, sleep is both profound and long, sometimes even absorbing a large portion of the day.

In *monomania*, sleep is generally broken or disturbed by hallucinations, and the patient in this state talks to himself and reveals the subject of his hallucination, which when awake he was studious to conceal. Among other objective symptoms of insanity, may be enumerated, neglect or eccentricity in dress, personal uncleanliness, a peculiar mousy smell, irregularity of appetite, alternations of excitement and depression, insensibility to vicissitudes of temperature. An inquiry into the history of the family, and the previous mode of life (habits, occupation, tastes and diseases, or accidents) of the patient, should also be made.

Epilepsy.

§ 81. The foregoing rules will apply with equal force to epilepsy, an intermittent disease of the brain, which is always a disqualification for military service.

The epileptic paroxysm is ushered in by a sudden loss of sensibility and consciousness, and a perversion of action in the muscles ordinarily under the control of the will. This perversion takes the form of clonic spasms, exhibiting violent and irregular contractions and extensions, accompanied by other unmistakable symptoms, which we shall presently describe.

The following differential diagnosis of *real* and *feigned* epilepsy will enable us to review, step by step, the course of the true disease; as well as the deviations therefrom, consequent upon simulation.

A. In real epilepsy, the paroxysm occurs *anywhere*, and the patient falls indiscriminately from heights, into water, the fire, on rocks, pavements, or the ground; while the simulator always selects some opportune time or place, so as to avoid injuring himself. Flexion of the thumbs upon the palms is one of the first symptoms to occur.

B. In real epilepsy, there is *an absolute loss of sensibility, with dilatation and immobility of the pupil.* Other phenomena present themselves with different degrees of distinctness, which, although unessential when considered separately, are yet of value in proportion as they approximate in resemblance.

C. In real epilepsy, the pupils remain immovable, while in the feigned disease, despite convulsions and contortions, the pupils always contract when a ray of bright light is thrown in upon them. In the true dis ease, the eyes are sometimes half-open, exhibiting only the sclerotica, and there is a convulsive twitching of the lids. At other times the eyes are wide open, with a vacant, haggard stare. This is the usual condition, towards the end of a paroxysm.

D. In real epilepsy, so complete is insensibility that neither the loudest sounds, nor the most penetrating and irritating odors, like ammonia and burning sulphur, nor tickling the soles of the feet, nor even cauterizing the surface, can provoke any sensation.

The foregoing operations generally suffice to evoke in simulators symptoms of painful perception, which at once reveal their deception. Even the threat, and the preparation of the actual cautery, made within their hearing, has sufficed sometimes to unmask simulation.

E. Among the accessory symptoms of real epilepsy are a red, bloated, contorted face, foaming at the mouth, and the state of the tongue—sometimes thrust out, sometimes seized between and bitten by the teeth. The appearance of the countenance cannot be imitated; foam produced by a piece of soap under the tongue is easily detected; and while thrusting out the tongue may be imitated, simulators are not apt to wound it. Again, in the true disease, respiration is embarrassed, the heart palpitates violently, the veins swell, and the pulse is small, feeble, and irregular; while in simulators it is full, quick, and bounding.

Again, in the true disease, the *thumbs* and wrists are flexed; if these are once extended, they remain so; while in simulators, these parts are no sooner extended than, as soon as pressure is removed, they flex them anew. In true epilepsy the skin is *clammy and cold*, in feigned cases it is hot.

F. At the termination of a true attack, the face loses its lividity, turns pale, wears a vacant, stupid look, while stertorous breathing sets in at the same time The pulse falls and becomes regular, respiration returns to its normal state, the patient pronounces some words with evident ignorance of what has transpired, complaining of headache, general fatigue, and finally recovers his senses with an imperious desire to sleep.

The surgeon should not allow himself to be deceived by either the force, violence, or duration of the convulsions, which malingerers will often prolong beyond the time usual in the true disease.

G. As the surgeon is not always present during attacks of epilepsy, he must analyze the external appearance of those in whom the disease is alleged or *sus-*

pected to exist, in order to discover such marks as it usually impresses upon the system, when become chronic.

In *chronic* epilepsy there may often be discovered some evidence of traumatic lesion, together with a special expression of countenance presenting one or more of the following features, viz.: timidity, shame, sadness, or stupidity. The upper eyelids droop, the head generally leans to one side or forward, the skin of the face is waxy and wrinkled, the pupils dilated, the voice husky, the veins swelled, the nostrils enlarged, the lips thickened, and the edges of both upper and lower incisors worn obliquely on corresponding sides.

After an attack of epilepsy, there will often be found contusions, and even wounds, made by the patient falling against something, or striking himself; and the tongue often shows traces of having been bitten, while the teeth are occasionally found injured.

H. Cold douches to the face, the introduction of snuff into the nostrils, and tickling either these or the soles of the feet, always produce manifestations of sensation in malingerers.

Whenever an application for a discharge on the ground of epilepsy is made, the soldier should be sent to the hospital for observation. The surgeon, or his assistants, can there easily satisfy themselves of the existence or simulation of the disease.

Epilepsy can also be concealed by a recruit, when it has as yet left no permanent marks upon the system. In such case the surgeon must seek elsewhere, than in the man himself, for proof of its existence, and public report is the best source to which to apply.

Alcoholic epilepsy, common among the intemperate,

is curable by proper treatment, and merits no special notice in this connection.*

Epileptic Vertigo.

§ 82. This is a modified form of epilepsy, in which the paroxysm is marked neither by convulsions, swelling of the face, nor foaming at the mouth. It consists in a sudden loss of sensation and consciousness, fixed stare with involuntary flow of saliva, muscular relaxation, with falling, or simply vacillation of the body. After the attack, which lasts only a few minutes, the patient resumes his occupations, unconscious of what has occurred. This form of epilepsy, which predisposes to grave lesions of the intellectual faculties, requires likewise that the recruit should be rejected and the soldier discharged.

* Percy and Laurent (Dict. des Sciences Medicales) mention the case of a Parisian beggar who was in the habit of feigning epilepsy, in order to provoke the sympathy of passers-by, and thus obtain their alms. The police suspecting the cheat, however, caused a straw bed to be placed near him, upon which, when the fit was next feigned, he threw himself in violent contortions; fire was thereupon immediately applied to each corner, when the beggar sprang to his feet, and ran away!

Another instance related by them, occurred in a young cavalry soldier, who feigned the disease so well, that even Percy was for awhile deceived. The foaming at the mouth, flexion of the thumbs, and insensibility were capitally counterfeited, and a discharge was about being granted; when the distinguished surgeon determined to make one trial, and this a crucial one, of the reality of the disease. Accordingly, the next time the fit came on, he approached the subject, examined him carefully, and then in a loud voice ordered the farrier to heat quickly a horseshoe red-hot, and apply it to the patient's posteriors. The moment the farrier was seen coming with his pincers and horseshoe in hand, and the assistants proceeded to take down the man's trousers, the better to apply this new argument *a posteriori*, the simulator rose upon his knees and confessed his fraud. He afterwards related to Baron Percy that his father had taught him the art of simulation, in which it would seem he had himself nearly become an adept.

Catalepsy.

§ 83. This is an intermittent disease of extreme rarity, and, like epilepsy, returns at irregular intervals. Its usual symptoms are a sudden loss of sensation and consciousness, with rigidity of the muscles; so that the body and limbs retain during the entire paroxysm the position they had at its invasion. It is easy to ascertain loss of sensation by the cold douche, prickings, and irritants. Muscular rigidity can, to a certain degree, be simulated, but it always wants that complete stiffness which is observed among most cataleptics. When the paroxysm is witnessed by the surgeon, he cannot long remain in doubt as to its real or feigned character; but in the absence of ocular proofs, public report must be questioned upon the subject. When the existence of this disease is fully established, in either a recruit or a soldier, rejection or discharge must follow.

Somnambulism.

§ 84. There are no objective symptoms short of ocular proof, by which surgeons can distinguish the existence of this peculiar habit. But when it is proved to be chronic, and of frequent recurrence in an individual, he should be rejected or discharged.

Chorea.

§ 85. Chorea consists in an irregular and involuntary movement of one or more muscles, or, in fact, of the whole muscular system. It is quite a common affection, is not easily feigned, and when exhibited in a chronic form in an adult, unfits him for the military service.

Barking, is a correlated manifestation of chorea, which results from a spasm of the levator muscles of the larynx and the diaphragm. This condition can only be imitated by the visible concurrence of all the respiratory muscles. True barking often continues for several days; when feigned, it is not prolonged beyond a few hours, as exhaustion compels the discovery of the cheat.

Delirium Tremens.

§ 86. This disease, which requires no description, is only a disqualification for the military service, when its attacks have been repeated, when the subject of them is still addicted to indulgence in intoxicating drinks, and when, from his age, there is little hope of reforming him, or re-establishing his health.

Nostalgia.

§ 87. Nostalgia, or *home-sickness*, although not in itself a disease, is yet a predisposing cause to diseases of a most serious character. It has no connection with *recruiting*, and gives rise only to the question of a discharge among soldiers already in the service. Most authors are agreed in recognizing three distinct stages.

A. The first stage, marked by sadness, unrest, taciturnity, and moodiness, with lassitude and debility, and a disposition to abstraction of mind and revery.

B. In the second stage, the eyes are red, swelled, and haggard; deep sighs are emitted, and involuntary tears shed. The complexion becomes wan, appetite fails, digestion is languid; both secretions and excretions are impaired; perspiration diminishes; headache sets in; the sleep is disturbed by dreams of home; respiration becomes embarrassed, the skin dry, and the pulse soft and languid. Towards night fever supervenes, strength diminishes, emaciation comes on, and with it the intellectual faculties become degraded and extinguished.

C. In the third stage, all the foregoing symptoms become intensified. There is insomnolence, stupor, delirium, prostration, fever, colliquative diarrhœa, and marasmus finally closes the scene.

In its early stages, a furlough, judiciously granted, will often suffice to restore the moral vigor of the young soldier. But when it has long resisted treatment, and gone so far as to produce sensible external lesions, such as emaciation, or structural changes in large organs, a discharge must, unquestionably, be granted.

SECTION XVII.

DISEASES OF THE EARS.

§ 88. Perfect hearing being essential to the discharge of the duties of a soldier, the surgeon will give particular care to the examination of the ears of the recruit.

Loss of the Pavilion of the Ear.

§ 89. Hearing is generally imperfect in persons who have lost the whole or a part of the pavilion of the ear (the office performed by this being to collect the waves of sound, and to direct them towards the external meatus). Nevertheless, there are exceptions to this rule; and cases have been known in which individuals, losing the entire pavilion, have still retained their hearing unimpaired. Still, as a deformity, this accident requires the rejection of the *recruit*, although when it occurs in a *soldier*, and is accompanied by no sensible impairment of hearing, it affords no sufficient ground for a compulsory discharge.

Atrophy, Hypertrophy, &c.

§ 90. Atrophy, or its opposite hypertrophy, extensive tumors, ulcers, chronic eczema, or adherence to the skull, of the pavilion, are always causes for rejecting a recruit, on account either of the impairment of hearing they produce, the obstacles they present to the head-dress, or the possible dangers they give rise to from aggravation. The same rule applies to soldiers asking a discharge, whenever these disorders are such as to baffle surgical skill.

External Meatus.

§ 91. The meatus auditorius, in its normal state, being oblique within and forward, and describing a curve, whose convexity is upwards, it becomes necessary, in order to explore it, to examine the ear under a bright light (sunlight is preferable), at the same time pulling the pavilion backward, to straighten the curve of the duct. In placing the eye directly before the opening, it is nearly always possible to see the tympanum, which presents an oblique and pearly surface. This examination can be made much more thoroughly with the *speculum auris.*

Obliteration, &c.

§ 92. Complete obliteration, contraction or deviation of the meatus, and fungous growths in its cavity, are lesions which justify the rejection of a recruit, or the discharge of a soldier. They cannot be feigned.

Polypi.

§ 93. Polypi of the external meatus, when deeply seated, are always disqualifications for military service, owing to the uncertainty which attends their treatment. Among soldiers, if they are small, have a slight pedicle, and are situated at the external orifice of the meatus, they can be extirpated, and unless they show a disposition to return, afford no necessary cause for a discharge. But in contrary conditions they are ineradicable, and form an absolute disqualification.

Foreign Bodies.

§ 94. Foreign and inoffensive bodies often find their way into the external meatus, remain there undiscovered by the person, and thus interfere with hearing by directly preventing the passage of sonorous vibrations. The accumulation of wax (*cerumen*) often occasions a similar result. Both the obstacle and the deafness, consequent upon it, can be easily removed.

Peas, elder-pith, pieces of bread-crumb, and other analogous bodies, surreptitiously introduced into the meatus, have been alleged as morbid growths, occasioning incurable obstructions, and, in consequence, deafness. But a critical examination of the passage will not fail to disclose the cheat. In the first place, the auditory duct is free and healthy up to the obstacle perceived, and an instrument striking upon this meets with nothing like an organic resistance. When pricked, no blood flows; when pressed, it sinks farther in, without any apparent resistance from a point of attachment, and, finally, a simple manipulation with the forceps, or a stream of warm water, insures its removal.

Perforation of the Tympanum.

§ 95. Perforation of the tympanum is shown by the blowing of air through the ear, when the nostrils and mouth are closed, during expiration. This condition does not necessarily produce deafness. Nevertheless, and although the hearing may still be good, it is best to reject the recruit, because perforation being always the result of violent inflammation or injury of the internal ear, and air being constantly admitted into its cavity, predisposes it to recurrent inflammations.

Among soldiers perforation of the tympanum does not necessarily justify a discharge, unless deafness has ensued, or other accidents due to inflammation of the internal ear.

The Middle Ear—Obstruction, Contraction, Obliteration.

§ 96. Obstruction, contraction, or obliteration of the eustachian tube, due either to inflammation, enlargement of adjoining parts, or hypertrophy of the tonsils, often produces impairment or loss of hearing. These alterations of structure can only be ascertained by sounding the tube or carefully examining the back part of the mouth. By reason of the uncertainty attending their treatment, they always require that the recruit should be rejected. But in soldiers it is always well to subject them to special treatment, in order to determine the curability or incurability of the disorder, before venturing to give a discharge.

The Internal Ear.

§ 97. Affections of the internal ear, such as acute or chronic otitis of the cavity of the tympanum, diseases of the small bones, inflammation of the cellular tissue and of the periosteum of the cavity of the tympanum, are only appreciable by rational symptoms; their seat excluding all direct means of observation.

Acute Otitis.

§ 98. Acute otitis reveals itself by dull, and at times pulsative pains, accompanied by uncomfortable humming and ringing in the ears. These pains extend either in the direction of the external ear or the eustachian tube; in the first instance, the patient instinctively seeks to compress the ear with his hand; in the second, a painful sensibility is experienced in the pharynx, which incommodes deglutition. These local manifestations soon become general, and are accompanied by headache, vertigo, fever, and insomnolence. To these conditions is usually added temporary deafness, of a more or less marked character. This disease, which is entirely amenable to treatment, does not justify the rejection of a recruit, unless its symptoms are of great intensity. Nor does it afford ground for a discharge in soldiers, since, when properly treated, it would either cease or pass into the chronic state.

Chronic Otitis.

§ 99. Chronic inflammation of the cavity of the tympanum, which may or may not follow the acute form of that disease, is particularly observed among persons subjected to constant humidity, such as the inhabitants of maritime countries, as also among lymphatic temperaments and those predisposed to scrofula. It produces an imperfect deafness, of variable intensity, and which appears to be controlled by atmospheric influences.

The patient hears better in dry than in wet weather, and his hearing is also affected according as the congestion of the tissues, together with the effusion of fluids, prevents the circulation of air between the eustachian tube and the cavity of the tympanum. The transparency of the drum is also often diminished.

In cases of this kind, and wherever it is evident that the phenomena described above are not the product of attempts at simulation, it is best to reject the recruit. While in soldiers if, after having undergone proper treatment, the disease still continues incurable, a discharge should be granted.

Purulent Discharges.

§ 100. When purulent discharges are solely confined to the external meatus, no cause for rejection presents itself; since it is generally a temporary affection, and often consecutive to typhoid fever or scarlatina. Nor would it justify a discharge, unless it had obstinately resisted all treatment. Purulent discharge from the external meatus is distinguished from that coming from the internal ear, by the absence of all signs of perforation of the tympanum (blowing air from the ear). But if the eustachian tube is either obliterated or obstructed, no air will escape and the origin of the discharge cannot be ascertained through this channel. In such cases we must explore the external ear with great care, employing at the same time the speculum or forceps.

Purulent discharges are sometimes feigned, by the introduction of honey into the external ear, of the greenish juice of herbs, and of tallow mixed with assafœtida, or old cheese ; but each of these substances has a special fetor which differs essentially from that of the pus—always strong smelling in itself—which the ears secrete. Sometimes pus itself is introduced, but this is easily detected by syringing the ear with warm water and afterwards wiping it dry.

A true purulent, fetid discharge is sometimes the result of an artificially produced otitis, through the action of topical irritants. It is of course difficult to obtain proof of this fact; but the simulator generally pays the penalty due to such deception, by the permanent injury entailed upon himself.

Purulent discharges may also be concealed by cleansing the external ear, just previous to the surgeon's examination. But in this case the appearance of the duct is white, humid, and as it were macerated and wholly deprived of wax; while in a state of health, it is always dry, yellowish-looking, and coated more or less with yellow or brownish wax of marked consistency.

Suppuration of the Mastoideal Cells.

§ 101. The mastoideal cells may be the seat of diffusive suppuration, arising from caries of the petrous portion of the temporal bone. In such case the integuments are œdematous, forming a hard, incompressible tumor which sometimes crackles under pressure. This formation adds to the severe pain usually present. This is a somewhat rare affection; but, being always serious in character, disqualifies a person absolutely for the military service.

Deafness.

§ 102. Deafness may result from various structural alterations, not discoverable on examination, or from a simple nervous affection without any visible alteration of parts. But long-subsisting deafness and the suspension of the relations to which hearing gives rise, impress upon the general appearance of the individual very characteristic signs. The truly deaf, whose intelligence is not at the same time impaired, exhibits in his features, in the expression of his countenance, and of his eyes a sort of interrogative attention which seeks to penetrate, through the motion of the speaker's lips, what is said to him. This demeanor, of difficult simulation, does not always exhibit itself to an equal degree; but it is always in contrast with the dull and stupid air assumed by the simulator, and which should always awaken attention.

The explosion of a percussion-cap or a simple clapping of the hands suffice to awaken the simulator. Threats, or harsh words, will induce either the pallor of fear in his countenance, or the glow of suppressed anger. No general method for surprising him can be given. The circumstances of each case must stimulate the sagacity of the surgeon and furnish him with the readiest means. As a rule the simplest expedients are the best, being the ones least expected by simulators. *Congenital* deafness is necessarily accompanied by dumbness, a fact to which the physiognomy of the person and public report generally certify. Yet deafness is one of those disqualifications for a soldier's life which is very often feigned. The belief that it only requires perfect self-control, that the structural changes of which it may be the result are deep-seated and inaccessible to exploration, lead men to undertake that which they conceive the surgeon has no means of confuting. And as a fact it must be confessed, that these cases often occasion great embarassment. Still, they must be explored whenever suspected, relying upon the ability of science to triumph in the end over deceit.

Whenever an alleged deaf man presents himself for examination, the first step to be taken is to thoroughly explore the pavilion of the ear, the opening and whole extent of the auditory duct, the tonsils, the pharynx, and the parts that are adjacent to the arches of the palate. Next ascertain whether any air enters into the cavity of the tympanum, and whether it does not escape through a perforation of this membrane. If in the course of this examination any obliterations, morbid growths, thickening of tissues, or tumors, compressing and obliterating the auditory passages are met with, the cause of the deafness is explained, and the recruit must be rejected. The same rule obtains when perforation of the tympanum is discovered (§ 95). It is safe to suspect a deaf man who asserts that he can hear nothing in however high a key, and however closely he is addressed.

In calling away attention from himself and gradually lowering the voice, proofs of modified hearing are often discovered. The vocation pursued by the person, will give an indirect clue to the real degree of hearing enjoyed by him. It must not be forgotten, in this connection, that a man may be deaf, and yet be able to perceive, by the shock imparted to the floor, the fall of a body near him, or perceive very shrill sounds, like those of a bell, while perfectly unable to hear loud and deep sounds. There are degrees too, in deafness, which must not be overlooked. By inquiring into the history of the recruit, proofs outside of physical exploration can thus be easily obtained of his infirmity.

Among soldiers applying for a discharge, it will be the fault of surgeons if they are not subjected to a thorough and prolonged examination, calculated to establish the fact of the disease beyond a doubt, before being declared incapacitated for military service.

Deafness may be concealed, on which account, every recruit should have some words addressed to him in a low tone of voice.*

* Dr. Casper (Handbuch der Gerichtlichen Medicin, tom. 1) gives the two following instances of feigned deafness:—

A female convicted of theft and imprisoned, complained that the dampness of her cell had rendered her deaf. Even when addressed in the loudest tones, she appeared not to hear. Suspecting her veracity, the Doctor pretended to believe her, and to prescribe for the disorder. And on one occasion, while visiting her, exclaimed aloud, "Good Heavens! there is *vermin* here!" and suddenly turning towards the prisoner, said in a very low voice, "Madame, you have a *louse* on your right sleeve!" The woman instantly turned, and examined her right arm, with a motion of evident disgust.

The next instance is that of an old woman who was tried for an assault upon a female with a sickle. The prisoner pretended to be sick, feeble, and completely deaf; and no amount of voice on the part of the Court sufficed to make her understand any thing. Casper was thereupon called in, who, from the bearing of the woman, at once suspected her of feigning. Approaching her ear, he shouted, "You are accused of having grievously wounded Mrs. Lemke." "It's a lie," replied the prisoner. "But," rejoined the Doctor, "Mrs. Lemke would not say so, were it not true; for"—suddenly dropping his voice into a whisper—"you know Mrs. Lemke is not a liar." "*She is a liar*," exclaimed the prisoner aloud, pushed by the spirit of revenge to gratify her hatred, even at the expense of exposing her own deception.

SECTION XVIII.

DISEASES OF THE FACE.

§ 103. The general aspect of the countenance usually indicates the alterations of which it is the seat. A single glance will often discover organic lesions, which are disqualifications for the military service. Thus, a hectic flush raises a presumption of phthisis; a straw-yellow tinge, that of the cancerous cachexy; while puffiness and infiltration point either to disease of the heart or kidney. Extreme deformity of feature or repulsiveness; atrophy of some portion of the face, or want of symmetry between its sides, may all form causes of rejection. Any thing, in fact, which is calculated to render the soldier uncompanionable or disgusting to his fellows, is a disqualification for the military service, most of whose duties are discharged in common.

Deformities and Exostosis of the Forehead.

§ 104. Excessive protuberance or deformity of the forehead is rare, but when it does occur, always forms a cause for rejection, on account of the obstacle it presents to the soldier's head-dress, which usually consists of some hard, unyielding fabric.

Exostoses seated upon the forehead are also causes for rejection, being for the most part dependent upon a bodily condition, which in itself constitutes a disability. When small, isolated, and situated upon other parts of the face, they are not necessarily causes for rejection.

Mutilations.

§ 105. Mutilations of the face from crushing of its bones, comminuted fractures (arising from attempts at suicide with fire-arms), are causes of accidental deformity, which generally incapacitate for the military service by reason of their extent, the obstacles to eating and speaking they occasion, and the aspect they impart to the physiognomy.

Tumors of various Kinds.

§ 106. The face is often the seat of various kinds of tumors, varieties of cysts (fatty, atheromatous, steatomatous, and bony), and erectile tumors and exostoses seem to select it of preference for their locality. When these affections are extensive, the recruit should be rejected; but when they appear in soldiers, no discharge should be granted until surgical treatment has proved unavailing.

Ulcers of the Face.

§ 107. Extensive ulcers of the face are causes for rejection but not of discharge, until surgical treatment has failed to cure them. But syphilitic ulcers, when not connected with a diseased constitutional habit (cachexy), nor of large size, are by reason of their curability, not a sufficient cause for rejection.

Fistulas.

§ 108. Fistulas of the face other than dental fistulas, are always a cause for rejection.

Cutaneous Diseases.

The face is the seat of many varieties of cutaneous

disease which, when chronic and extensive, or of contagious character, afford a cause for rejection. For example, lupus, sycosis, and cutaneous cancer.

Neuralgia.

§ 109. Facial neuralgia, or *Tic Douloureux* is a cause for rejection, whenever it has left external signs of its effects. When occurring in a soldier, no discharge should be granted until treatment has proved unsuccessful.

Paralysis.

§ 110. Partial paralysis of one side of the face may arise from trivial and temporary causes. The cause being first ascertained, the surgeon can then express a becoming opinion in the premises. Before discharging a soldier on this account resort should be had to treatment, in order to determine the question of its curability.

Facial hemiplegia is often symptomatic of serious cerebral disorder; in which case no doubt can be entertained as to the necessity of a rejection; but it is also frequently inflammatory (railroad paralysis) or syphilitic in character, and being then generally curable, does not justify either rejection or discharge.

SECTION XIX.

DISEASES OF THE EYE.

§ 111. The eyes, no less indispensable to the soldier than the ears, may be the seat of many forms of disease, manifesting themselves either in the ball, the lids, or the lachrymal passages, and alike disqualifying the recruit for military service. Some of these diseases may be feigned, others artificially produced, or concealed.

The methodical examination of the eye requires for its execution particular conditions. There must be a sufficiency of light, either natural or artificial, to enable the observer to appreciate the external condition of the eye, its size, color, secretions, and the aspect of the pupil.

Touch is also necessary to ascertain the consistence of the organ, which may vary with the health, or to determine whether the eye is natural or artificial.

The examination when made with the unassisted eye should be had under different aspects, viz.: with direct or oblique light, and sometimes with artificial light. Certain instruments also facilitate this examination. A magnifying glass brings into clearer view the external parts, such as the cornea, iris and crystalline lens, while spectacles, either convex or concave, serve to discover the existence of myopia, presbyopia, and hypermetropia.

The ophthalmoscope is indispensable for a critical examination of the internal structure of the eye, and may bring to light forms of disease which cannot otherwise be distinguished.

DISEASES OF THE BALL OF THE EYE.

Mechanical Lesions.

§ 112. Any abnormal conditions of the ball of the eye, either in its position, direction, form, consistence, or in the proportion between its parts, and resulting from disease or external violence, may afford a cause for rejection, whenever they occasion disturbances of the sight. Such results are often consecutive to mechanical injuries, and vary with each particular case.

Foreign Bodies.

§ 113. The examining surgèon should be careful to scrutinize cases of loss or impairment of sight, said to be due to foreign bodies in the eye. Internal ophthalmia of one eye, due to the presence of a foreign body, such as a fragment of percussion cap, should always constitute a cause for rejection or discharge, particularly if the sight of the fellow-organ be impaired. Extirpation of a sightless and inflamed left eye, may save the fellow-organ and justify the refusal of a discharge.

Exophthalmos.

§ 114. Protrusion of the eye may be congenital or acquired. In such cases the eye is thrust out of its orbit by a cause acting from behind and within, and forms what is known as exophthalmos. This disease may be either idiopathic, or symptomatic of local lesions, or of some general constitutional habit attended with impairment of sight; it always forms a cause for rejection. When it occurs in a soldier, he should first undergo treatment to test its curability, before receiving a discharge.

Atrophy.

§ 115. Atrophy of the eye may result from various structural alterations, and always constitutes a disqualification for military service.

Ophthalmia.

§ 116. A vague term, but generally restricted to inflammatory affections of the ocular and palpebral conjunctiva, and of the tarsal edges. The acute forms of the disease should not of themselves be considered a cause for rejection or discharge. The chronic forms, especially when characterized by granular roughness of the palpebral conjunctiva, or vasculo-nebulous or ulcerated cornea, disqualify the patient for military service. But the examining surgeon must satisfy himself of the genuine character of the lesions, so as to avoid imposture.

Men have been known to present themselves suffering from alleged chronic ophthalmia, in whom the eyelashes had been purposely extracted, and the edges of the lids cauterized. But in such cases a strict watch and the lapse of time will suffice to unmask the deception.

If the means employed by the simulator have been continued for a long time, the lesions induced may be of such a nature as to justify a rejection or discharge. The surgeon will readily discover the agents, chemical or otherwise, employed to produce the disease. Chronic conjunctivitis, accompanied by granular lids, or opacities of the cornea, invariably requires rejection or discharge.

Glaucoma.

§ 117. Glaucoma is generally considered to be a disease of the choroid membrane with serous effusion. When confirmed, its external manifestations are usually well marked by a glassy appearance of the cornea, an unyielding hardness of the eye-ball, as if a billiard ball were beneath the lids, and dilatation of the pupil. The patient suffers more or less pain and sees iridescent hues; an increasing presbyopia and limitation of the visual field are also very significant. This disease is a cause for rejection and discharge. The opthalmoscopic appearances are marked, and should be sought for in every case.

Diseases of the Cornea.

§ 118. Conical cornea, extreme prominence or transparent staphyloma of the cornea, which seriously impairs the sight constitutes a disqualification for military service.

Wounds and Foreign Bodies.

§ 119. Wounds of the cornea resulting from external violence, or the presence of a foreign body are of importance according to their effect upon vision.

Keratitis.

§ 120. Whether acute or chronic is always a cause for rejection, since it rarely fails to destroy the transparency of the cornea, and thus to impair sight.

Ulcerations.

§ 121. Ulcers of the cornea are of variable importance, according to their position and depth. If the ulceration be superficial, narrow, and situated out of the field of vision, it is not a disqualification for military service. But if it be deep and extensive, it affords a cause for rejection. Discharges to soldiers should be granted only after treatment has proved unavailing.

Opacities.

§ 122. Opacities upon the cornea afford no cause for rejection, unless situated before the pupil, or accompanied by granular lids.

Staphyloma.

§ 123. Staphyloma of the cornea interfering more or less with vision, and always of doubtful cure, is an absolute cause for rejection or discharge.

Astigmatism.

§ 124. Astigmatism, whether due to aberration in the curve of the cornea or lens, should be a cause of rejection or discharge.

DISEASES OF THE IRIS.

Loss of Color.

§ 125. The iris at times loses somewhat of its color, or exhibits a difference in color between the two eyes. This state, which is usually congenital, does not generally impair the perfection of vision, except in albinoes. Sometimes, however, loss of color in the iris may lead to the suspicion of old iritis. We must then ascertain whether adhesions exist between the iris and lens impairing sight. The mobility of the iris may be ascertained by opening and closing the eyelids in a good light, or by the use of some agent, as belladonna or atropine.

Congenital Fissures.—Lacerations.

§ 126. Congenital fissures of the iris are generally unimportant, but lacerations or perforations require to be considered according to their extent and effects upon vision.

Absence of the Iris.

§ 127. Absence of the iris in either eye, is a cause for rejection.

Atresia.

§ 128. Complete closure of the pupil is a cause for rejection or discharge.

Dilatation of the Pupil.

§ 129. Dilatation of the pupil, when slight, is not incompatible with perfect vision. When excessive and permanent, it affords a cause for rejection. The surgeon should be on his guard against this state, artificially produced by specific substances.

Detachment.

§ 130. The iris may be detached from the ciliary ligament, and thus an artificial pupil be produced. When the detachment is slight, it has no effect upon vision. Sometimes this membrane is caught in a scar of the cornea, producing a condition which may be slight and inconsequential in its effects upon vision, or cause a serious impairment of it. The surgeon must judge of these diversities of effect in forming an opinion.

Tremor of the iris may indicate softening of the vitreous humor or luxation of the crystalline lens, and as it causes a serious impairment of vision, is a disqualification for military service. The ophthalmoscope should be used to assist in deciding the character of a given case, and the vision should be accurately tested for amblyopia.

Iritis.

§ 131. Inflammation of the iris appears under three different forms, viz.: *traumatic*, *syphilitic*, and *rheumatic*, each of which presents characteristic local symptoms. These diseases are all causes for rejection when they are well marked, not only on account of their intensity, but of their very nature. The syphilitic form, by far the most common, is generally accompanied by constitutional symptoms. It should invariably secure rejection, as it furnishes one of the clearest evidences of constitutional syphilis; it should also induce discharge from service.

Diseases of the Sclerotic.

§ 132. Special diseases of the sclerotic are rare. The only one deserving mention here is a species of atrophy or thinning of this membrane, which is characterized by a dark discoloration, due to the exposure of the pigment color of the choroid. This condition is a disqualification for military service.

Diseases of the Crystalline Lens and of its Capsule.

§ 133. Dislocation of the crystalline lens is of rare occurrence. When present and from whatever cause arising, whether traumatic or spontaneous, whether the lens be opaque or transparent, reducible or irreducible, it is always a cause for rejection or discharge.

Cataract.

§ 134. Cataract, which should always occasion either rejection or discharge, is, when well advanced, appreciable by the naked eye. Yet it may be necessary in certain incipient cases to resort to a magnifying-glass, or to oblique illumination. This last-named operation consists in examining the pupil by artificial light, which has been made to traverse a convex lens of about two inches focus. The observer will find it convenient to stand behind and above the head of the person inspected, so as to get the light reflected from the crystalline lens. By this process adhesions of the iris to the capsule of the lens may be seen; delicate ulcerations of the cornea, and even foreign bodies, should any happen to be attached to the surface, or entangled in the substance of the cornea, may also be detected. No examination for cataract can be complete, however, without the use of the ophthalmoscope, the pupil having been previously dilated by belladonna or atropine.

Diseases of the Internal Parts of the Eye,

CONTINUED.

§ 135. The progress of ophthalmoscopy has enabled us to ascertain that amaurosis is not the consequence of a single and always the same lesion, but may result from many diseases differing no less in their nature than in their locality.

All these diseases present as their characteristic sign, an impairment of vision (amblyopia) or loss of sight (amaurosis), in one or both eyes, without exhibiting to the naked eye any obstacle, preventing the access of light to the retina.

Amaurosis, having its origin in the ball of the eye or optic nerve, is nearly always discoverable by the ophthalmoscope. Negative indications presented by this instrument will turn the attention of the surgeon to the brain or more remote portions of the body. A careful study of the rational symptoms of brain disease will generally result in such a diagnosis as will eliminate all doubt of the propriety of rejection or discharge.

In deep affections of the eye accompanied by photophobia the employment of the ophthalmoscope requires caution. A method of examination which should never be neglected is that of producing phosphenes.* This may be done by placing the subject in a darkened room, and when the eyelids are partially closed applying quick and interrupted pressure upon the eyeball.

Amaurosis dependent upon the Optic Nerve—Atrophy.—Hyperœmia.—Choroid Congestion.—Apoplexy, or Softening.

§ 136. Diseases of the optic nerve can only be recognized by the aid of the ophthalmoscope. Its atrophy, a frequent cause of amaurosis, and which is often complicated with cerebral amaurosis, is indicated by a glittering, pearly whiteness, and the smallness of the branches of the retinal arteries. In its normal state it presents a pale, pinkish-yellow appearance.

All diseases of the deep-seated parts of the eye, whether producing loss of sight, or only weakness, whether existing in one eye or in both, are causes for rejection or discharge.

At the same time it must not be forgotten, that amaurosis is one of those diseases the existence of which is most often *feigned.*

Having learned that the diseases comprehended under this designation are slow in their progress, and that they present no very characteristic objective symptoms at the outset, the malingerer readily asserts that his sight is either weak, or that he does not see at all.

In most instances the ophthalmoscope will detect the deception; failing to do so, there are other tests known to art by which all doubt can be removed, such as

* Phosphenes are luminous circles produced by forcible compression of the eyeball, for the purpose of testing retinal sensibility.

employing prismatic glasses to produce double images, etc. The latter expedient can be so managed as to detect many forms of imposture. For instance, a man may allege that he cannot see with one eye. Take him into a dark room, apply prismatic glasses, and produce a lighted candle; of course he says he sees two lights, and the deception is detected. This experiment may be so varied as to render imposture very difficult, if not impossible.

The patient's recital of his own case will contribute much towards assisting the surgeon's examination. You should also observe the comparative condition of the pupils, whether one is larger than the other, and whether it has the power of contraction when the fellow-eye is darkened. If he asserts it to be of long standing, the manifestations ought to be deeply marked.

Differential Diagnosis of Blindness from Amaurosis and from Cataract.

§ 137. Blindness resulting from amaurosis impresses upon the countenance an entirely different character from that arising from cataract. There need therefore be no difficulty in distinguishing them. The amaurotic subject carries his head high, and opens his eyes widely, in order to collect as much light as possible within the pupil, and thus stimulate whatever sensibility still remains in the retina. The subject of cataract, on the contrary, bows his head and inclines it in different directions, seeking for the position most favorable to the transmission of light between the iris and the opaque lens.

Amaurosis and cataract are not the only causes of loss of sight; but from whatever source this latter may originate, and whether partial or complete in its nature, it always constitutes an absolute disqualification for military service.

IMPAIRMENT OF SIGHT.

Myopia (Near-sightedness).

§ 138. Near-sightedness cannot be recognized with certainty by external inspection of the eye alone. The use of glasses, and of the ophthalmoscope, is requisite to establish the diagnosis. If the subject, with double concave glasses of six-inch focus before his eyes, can read fine type (pearl) when held at a distance of less than six inches, no doubt can be entertained of his disability for military service. A less degree of myopia, especially when accompanied by posterior staphyloma, pigment maceration of the choroid, or floating bodies in the vitreous, may also justify his rejection.

In case the subject is unable to read, a simple and very conclusive test is that of successively applying various glasses for short-sightedness, and also plain glasses before his eyes without allowing him to examine them previously. The simulator cannot distinguish beforehand those with which it would be impossible for him to read, were he really near-sighted.

The existence of posterior staphyloma will be revealed by the use of the ophthalmoscope, and may always be suspected when the myopia is progressive, and characterized by any marked inequality in the sensibility of the retinal field.

Presbyopia.

§ 139. Presbyopia, or long sightedness is rarely encountered by the examining surgeon, for it is a disorder belonging to middle or old age. Convex glasses are its proper test, but in order to justify rejection, it should exist to a high degree. Even among old soldiers it is not a cause for discharge.

Hypermetropia.

Hypermetropia may exist at any age, and, if exceeding $\frac{1}{15}$, should cause rejection. The necessity of correcting this abnormity by the constant use of lenses is incompatible with the duties of a soldier.

Hemiopia (Partial Sight).

§ 140. In hemiopia the sight is limited to a part only of the object viewed. This state most frequently depends upon detachment of the retina, and other affections of the posterior tunics of the eye, as well as, in some instances, upon changes in the brain.

Diplopia (Double Sight).

§ 141. Diplopia, whether monocular or binocular generally results from derangement of the parallelism of the visual axes, and most often originates in muscular paralysis. The nature of the diplopia will depend of course upon the muscle or muscles at fault, and can only be decided by a careful study of each case, with the assistance of a slide of colored glass and a lighted candle in a darkened room.

Well marked diplopia is always a cause for rejection. In a soldier it may be curable and then not justify a discharge until the efficient cause has been ascertained to be of a nature unsusceptible of cure.

Pseudoblepsia (False Vision).

§ 142. Pseudoblepsia is an affection in which false objects appear before the sight; such, for example, as the motes termed *muscæ volitantes.* It is often the first stage of amaurosis.

The foregoing affections reveal themselves by no external sign, yet in certain cases much valuable information may be obtained by the ophthalmoscope. They require that the recruit be rejected, if their cause depends upon serious lesions of tissue. But they justify a discharge only if springing from progressive, structural changes.

Photophobia (Intolerance of Light).

§ 143. This condition is symptomatic of diseases which often may, but which do not necessarily, justify either a rejection or discharge. It may depend upon some curable disease of the conjunctiva or cornea, and therefore render a discharge from service improper; or it may supervene upon some fever or blood disease, and gradually subside as convalescence progresses. A displaced eye lash may be the only cause for its presence.

Hemeralopia (Night-Blindness).

§ 144. In hemeralopia the person sees clearly during the day and becomes blind during the night. At sunset surrounding objects begin to be covered by a grayish veil; he scarcely sees them, or not at all, when illuminated by an artificial light amply sufficient for bystanders; and he sees even less clearly by moonlight. At day-break sight returns, and again continues in its normal state until sunset. It may be consequent upon cerebral congestion, certain intestinal diseases, scurvy, and pernicious fevers. There is no test by which its genuine character can be determined; generally the ophthalmoscope reveals marked choroidal congestion of a passive character.

Nyctalopia (Day-Blindness).

§ 145. Nyctalopia, the opposite condition of the foregoing disease, is of rather rare occurrence. In this disorder the person sees objects only dimly or not at all during the day, or when they are illuminated; while in a dark place at evening, or during the ordinary darkness of night, he sees them very well.

Both the foregoing diseases justify the rejection or discharge of an individual.

DISEASES OF THE CONJUNCTIVA.

Ecchymoses.

§ 146. Care must be taken not to confound ecchymoses of the conjunctiva with inflammation of that membrane, the ordinary form in which ophthalmia manifests itself. The former may result from external violence and be of no importance, or, on the other hand, they may indicate a condition of plethora or a scorbutic cachexy. The plethoric congestion may be the result of temporary excitement, while scorbutic ecchymoses constitute a serious condition, requiring rejection of the recruit, by reason of the impairment of constitution which they indicate.

Chemosis (Elevation of the Conjunctiva above the Cornea).

§ 147. Chemosis may be a cause for rejection, if it be

severe and threaten the integrity of the cornea. The value of this condition must depend, in a great measure, upon the nature of the disease of which it is a symptom.

Cysts.

§ 148. Cysts and fibrous tumors of the conjunctiva are generally of small size and easily curable. They however require the rejection of a party, if they present themselves in the vicinity of the cornea and encroach upon it.

Pannus.

§ 149. Pannus is always an absolute disqualification for military service.

Pterygion is a varicose, pyramidal shaped development of the vessels of the conjunctiva, whose base rests upon the sclerotic, and whose summit extends towards the centre of the cornea. Unless obstructing vision, pterygion is not a cause either for rejection or discharge.

Xerosis (Dry Ophthalmia).

§ 150. Xerosis or dryness of the conjunctiva is a rare disease and always a cause for rejection or discharge.

DISEASES OF THE ORBIT.

Deformities.

§ 151. Deformities of the orbit are extremely rare, and, in the majority of instances, are complicated with diseased conditions which interfere with sight. Sometimes a narrowness or species of atrophy of this cavity is met with, which may be a cause for rejection.

Fractures.

§ 152. Fractures, loss of substance, and cicatrices are the only mechanical lesions of the orbit requiring notice. In determining the question of disability, the surgeon must consider the extent of the lesion present, or the loss of substance ensuing.

Foreign Bodies.

§ 153. Foreign bodies may be lodged in the orbit and occasion inflammations, abscess, ostitis, caries, and necrosis.

Tumors.

§ 154. Various kinds of tumors, although of rare occurrence, develop themselves within this cavity, having their seat either external to, or within its walls, and producing exophthalmos. Such are abscesses, cysts, fatty and erectile tumors, exostoses, or aneurism. These always form causes for rejection, and sometimes for discharge.

DISEASES OF THE MUSCLES OF THE EYE.

Strabismus.

§ 155. Strabismus is the consequence of functional disorder of the nerves, or of cerebral disease. It is simple or double, convergent or divergent, primitive or consecutive to tenotomy. Permanent, fixed strabismus of the right eye is always a disqualification for military service, by reason of the deviation in this organ which it causes, and the impairment in functional tone which inevitably precedes or follows it.

Strabismus may be feigned, but then it is slight and subject to variation.

Before expressing any opinion in the premises, the surgeon should satisfy himself that the deviation is fixed and permanent.

Feigned strabismus may be detected by awaking the subject from sleep. Under this test, the lids in opening will exhibit the eyeballs in their normal state of parallelism; the same proof may also be obtained by examining the eyes when the person is asleep.

When the party is awake, a great and sudden surprise practised upon him, will often be sufficient to make him forget the part he is acting; or in order to discover the cheat, he may be compelled to follow with his eyes an object slowly passed before them. Among simulators strabismus is commonly binocular, it is always convergent. Generally speaking, the fatigue resulting from the continued voluntary contraction of the muscles of the ball of the eye, puts an end of itself to the deception, and this may also be discovered by placing the party aside, and under rigorous supervision for a short time.

When the strabismus unites the two conditions of permanence and fixedness, there is always a tendency to retraction of the motor muscles of the eye, particularly of the internal rectus muscle, and the deviation usually increases progressively, together with the impairment of sight. A somewhat frequent form of strabismus observed is that known as alternating-convergent.

Nystagmus.

§ 156. The muscles of the eye are at times the seat of a spasmodic contraction, of variable intensity, termed nystagmus, which is sometimes a symptom of disease of the brain.

This condition is accompanied by a sensible diminution of sight and requires rejection. It may be feigned, but a critical examination soon exposes the cheat. In real nystagmus the motion of the eyes is extremely rapid, with increased vibrations and deviations when a distant object is viewed, and diminishing markedly, or ceasing, when a nearer one is looked at; hence the motion is usually lessened in reading. In true nystagmus there is almost invariably a tendency to bring objects looked at close to the eye. This disease always requires the rejection or discharge of its subject, since it is invariably associated with cataract or retino-chorodial disease.

DISEASES OF THE EYELIDS.

Deformities.

§ 157. Absence or atrophy of the lids is extremely rare, but always a disqualification for military service.

Adhesions.

§ 158. Adhesions of the lids, either between themselves (ankyloblepharon) or to the ball of the eye (symblepharon),and the lesions following them—inversion (entropion), or eversion (ectropion)—are causes for rejection, whenever the adhesions are sufficiently extensive to impair the sight or induce irritability of the eyes ; but no discharge should be granted until treatment has proved unavailing.

Trichiasis.

§ 159. Inversion of the eyelashes (trichiasis), or their abnormal development and direction, (distichiasis), or their entire loss, exposes the eye to inflammation and is a cause for rejection. Trichiasis may be treated successfully : hence the subject of discharge need not be alluded to in this connection.

Wounds.

§ 160. Wounds of the eyelids, cicatrices, chronic inflammations, hypertrophy, encysted or other tumors, as well as ulcers, are either compatible with the discharge of military duties, or else require rejection of the recruit, according to their extent and severity. Many of these lesions may be cured by methodical treatment, or a slight surgical operation; as, for example, encysted tumors, abnormal adhesions, &c.: hence, these lesions are less a cause for discharge than for rejection.

Blepharospasm.

§ 161. Blepharospasm is an affection marked by involuntary and convulsive movements of the eyelids, alternating with intervals of repose. It is always a cause for rejection.

Spasm of the eyelids may be feigned by the simple operation of the will, or produced by the momentary introduction of a foreign body beneath the eyelids. In the first instance, the party must be observed when his attention is called away and excited by others; or if the introduction of a foreign body is its cause, careful scrutiny will exhibit more redness of the conjunctiva and weeping than in the real disease. Moreover, there will be noticed rather a predominant contraction of the orbicular muscle than a regular, yet instantaneous, alternation in the closing and opening of the eyelids.

This disorder must not be confounded with habitual winking, a condition generally speaking, of little importance, and which would require rejection only when very severe and dependent upon some incurable lesions of the palpebral conjunctiva, or deformity of the edges of the eyelids.

Hordeolum.

§ 162. The ordinary stye can never deceive the surgeon, nor cause itself to be mistaken for any thing serious.

Granulations.

§ 163. Granulations of the eyelids may be either the cause, or the consequence of inflammation. They justify rejection or discharge whenever well marked. Yielding very slowly to treatment, they become formidable by reason of their contagiousness and disastrous influence upon the health, and transparency, of the cornea. Even when not of the contagious variety, they lead the way by changes in the shape of the eyelids to trichiasis or distichiasis, and thus may impair the health and transparency of the cornea after all roughness of the palpebral conjunctiva has disappeared. A person having once had granular lids, is subject to a recurrence of the disease.

Paralysis.

§ 164. The eyelids may lose their power of performing either of the functions of *opening* or *closing*, owing to either contraction of the levator palpebræ superioris, or paralysis of the orbicular muscle, or ptosis, or spasm of the orbicularis.

Inability to close the Eye.

§ 165. Tonic contraction of the levator muscle is rare and symptomatic of nervous disease, which forms of itself a cause for rejection. Paralysis of the orbicular muscle never exists without more or less paralysis in other branches of the facial nerve. It forms a disqualification for the military service, particularly when of long standing. It may be symptomatic of constitutional disease of a curable character, and should, therefore, have the benefit of appropriate treatment, before occasioning discharge from service.

Occlusion.

§ 166. Occlusion may arise from paralysis of the levator muscie, or adhesions between the eyelids, or the eyelids and eyeball.

This disorder may at times be temporary, and owing to inflammatory or sanguineous tumefaction of the eyelids, or adjoining tissues, to erysipelas, eczema, or erythema. The ptosis should then disappear with its temporary cause. But if there be ptosis accompanied by flaccidity, and slight œdema of the cellular tissue, if the eyelid falls as soon as raised, or slowly settles down into its former position, without any other disease being present in its vicinity, the party must be rejected.

Ptosis is often accompanied by diplopia, divergent strabismus and mydriasis, and slight protrusion of the ball of the eye, all indicating paralysis of the third pair. In closely scrutinizing the eye, the loss of power in the muscles involved may be detected. The method of studying the double images will occur to any one familiar with modern opthalmology. The slide of colored glass, the candle in the darkened room, &c. This condition furnishes a cause both for rejection and discharge.

Holding the lid down and compressed for some time may produce a temporary inertia of the part, and if watery emollient applications have been made to it, a slight œdema supervenes, which, by its weight and tension, tends in turn to keep the lid down. This method of feigning ptosis has often been tried. The cheat can be readily exposed by slightly pinching the eyelid with the fingers or forceps into a fold. The party is then required to look up strongly with both eyes; immediately, the superior rectus muscle which receives its innervation from the same branch as the levator palpebræ superioris, carries the eye up and the lid follows instinctively from harmony of action; it is then also seen that there is neither dilatation of the pupil, nor divergent strabismus. Were the paralysis real, the eye could not be carried up under the lid, lifted by the fingers, and the eyelid could not raise itself. Even if some specific substance had been introduced into the eye for the purpose of dilating the pupil, the cheat could still be discovered in the absence of strabismus, for in this particular instance mydriasis could not well exist without strabismus.

DISEASES OF THE LACHRYMAL PASSAGES.

Tumefaction of the Lachrymal Gland.

§ 167. Each of the various parts constituting the lachrymal passages, may be the seat of some disqualifying disease.

At the external angle of the eye, the swollen lachrymal gland is occasionally, though rarely, seen uplifting the superior eyelid, constituting an external projection, pushing the eyeball inward, downward, and towards the nose, and even outside of the orbit, which produces a sufficient disturbance in the axis of vision to impair the sight. This disease dependent upon chronic inflammation or degeneration of the gland, and which can be neither feigned nor concealed, is an absolute disqualification for military service. In soldiers, although the tumor may be removed, particularly in the early stages of the disease, subsequent discharge is generally inevitable. The suppression of tears, which is owing for the most part to the extirpation of this, their secreting gland, exposes the eye to frequent causes of inflammation, not only by depriving it of continual lubrication, which neither the moisture of the conjunctiva, nor the secretions of the meibomian glands can replace, but also of the means of ridding itself, by super-secretion, of foreign bodies, dust for example, accidentally lodging between the eye ball and the lids.

Epiphora.

§ 168. An opposite condition to the foregoing is that of the superabundant secretion of tears, provoked by the slightest exciting cause, overflowing the eyes and spreading upon the cheeks. This is often a disqualification for military service, on account of the permanent irritation which results from it, and more particularly by reason of the annoyance and fatigue to the sight, produced by the new refraction, to which the rays of light are subjected before entering the pupil. This disease is generally the consequence of various forms of lesion which it becomes necessary to discover, since it is upon the lesion itself, rather than its result, that the surgeon must found his decision. Ordinarily it is easy to distinguish the slow and regular epiphora, occasioned by old and permanent lesions, from temporary epiphora, which might, for purposes of simulation, be excited by topical irritants. So also epiphora may be accidental and momentary, and arise from various unimportant causes.

Destruction, Obliteration of the Puncta Lachrymalia.

§ 169. Destruction of the puncta lachrymalia, fortunately a very rare thing, is a cause for rejection or discharge.

Partial occlusion of the puncta and of the lachrymal passages, does not in itself constitute a cause of incapacity. Congenital obliteration would alone constitute such a cause, but this is extremely rare. Partial occlusion by inflammation or obstruction is frequent enough, but generally curable.

Deviation of the Puncta and Lachrymal Ducts.

§ 170. Deviation of the puncta and lachrymal ducts, which may be the result of chronic thickening of the surrounding conjunctiva, of a tumor developed in that region, or of an eversion of the lower lid, produced by loss of substance, when sufficiently advanced to interfere with their functional activity, is always a cause for rejection, but not of discharge, for it is often susceptible of radical cure.

Lachrymal Tumor and Fistula.

§ 171. Lachrymal tumor and fistula, being different degrees of a similar disease, are always a cause for rejection, but only accidentally so, of a discharge. They result from inflammation of the canal and tear-sac, scrofula, syphilis, or wounds.

In order to distinguish the tumor, it suffices, if the surgeon is not already convinced by the coincidence of continual epiphora with distention of the lachrymal sac, to press this latter for the purpose of causing the contained fluid to exude through the puncta; when the puncta are closed by inflammatory swelling, the diagnosis must rest upon the observer's knowledge of the anatomy of the parts. In fistula the escape of tears through the ulceration situated over the sac, leaves no room for doubt.

Lachrymal tumor may result from acute inflammation of the canal and be cured by a simple treatment. It should not be a cause for rejection if the patient is otherwise healthy, but if dependent upon scrofula, syphilis, or a wound, rejection of the party must follow as a consequence.

Fistula lachrymalis can neither be feigned nor concealed; a clumsy mode of simulation might be practised by blowing air under the skin, but this accidental emphysema could hardly deceive the surgeon.

Chronic inflammation of the lachrymal sac, with disorganization of the sac walls and membranous lining of the nasal ducts, does not necessarily demand discharge, though they should preclude admission into the service. It has been demonstrated by large experience, that obliteration of the sac by the actual or potential cautery may be so effected as to restore the soldier to usefulness. Particularly is this the case when among soldiers the disease is confined to the left eye, and not due to scrofula or syphilis, or complicated by caries of the bony parts or confirmed ozæna.

Diseases of the Lachrymal Caruncle.

§ 172. The lachrymal caruncle is at times the seat of a soft excrescence of a red, livid hue, which, at first trifling, is liable to acquire a large size. The intervention of this tumor, or *encanthis*, between the commissure of the eyelids, which is thereby necessarily kept stretched, keeps up a chronic conjunctivitis and often produces epipho ra, by everting the orifices of the lachrymal ducts. Encanthis may assume a cancerous, fungous, or calculous character, in which conditions it always constitutes a disqualification for military service. Even when of a benign character, it is a cause for rejection, for it is only curable by extirpation ; but in soldiers it justifies a discharge only when its volume forbids its removal, or when after such operation, there remains some serious disorder, such as granular lids, epiphora, or eversion of the eyelid.

The lachrymal caruncle may be wanting, which is a rare thing; but this would justify neither a rejection nor a discharge.

SECTION XX.

DISEASES OF THE NOSE AND NASAL FOSSÆ.

§ 173. Examinations of the nose by the sight and touch are usually sufficient for the purpose of discovering its diseases; the sense of smell may also be used, together with the blunt probe, or catheter, employed in diseases of the nasal passages.

Deformities.

§ 174. Deformities of the nose to the extent of sensibly hindering either respiration or speech, and which may be congenital, or the result of fractures, of cicatrices consequent upon wounds, of burns, a rhinoplastic operation, or a state of permanent congestion, and producing either partial or complete loss of the nose, or its atrophy, hypertrophy, crookedness, flattening, or a crushing of its bridge—whenever these are of an extreme character, all form causes for rejection.

Herpetic Affections.

§ 175. The nose is the chief seat, and often the starting point of two herpetic diseases, which generally spread themselves over other parts of the face, and occasion more or less serious alterations. These are *lupus exedens*, already described by us; and *acnea rosacea*, a rare affection among the young, and which is distinguishable by its varying deep-red color. It attacks successively the cheeks and the forehead, which become thereby tumefied and deformed, as well as the nose. Its appearance is hideous and repulsive, and its cure always long and uncertain. These two diseases are absolute causes for rejection or discharge.

Obliteration of the Nostrils.

§ 176. Obliteration of the nostrils is very rare, and may result from hypertrophy of the cartilage.

Burns also sometimes occasion narrowing of these cavities, to the extent of impeding respiration. All such cases constitute an absolute disqualification for the military service.

Perforation of the Septum.—Foreign Bodies.

§ 177. Perforation of the dividing cartilage, or septum, is not incompatible with the discharge of military duties. The same rule will apply to foreign bodies, voluntarily or accidentally introduced into the nostrils, unless they have induced serious lesions.

Epistaxis.

§ 178. Habitual epistaxis, which may easily be feigned, is not a disqualification, unless it springs from a diseased condition of body.

Chronic Coryza.

§ 179. The pituitary membrane may be the seat of chronic inflammation, a condition which does not necessarily disqualify a recruit for service, unless it be so aggravated as to impede respiration. This condition is liable at times to be mistaken for polypus.

Polypus.

§ 180. Polypi which are of most frequent occurrence in the nasal fossæ, are absolute causes of disqualification in a recruit. Many of these polypi are in their nature recurrent, while others, though more rarely, tend to degenerate into cancer. When occurring in newly enlisted soldiers, no discharge should be granted, until the obstinacy of their recurrence plainly indicates their incurability.

Attempts at simulation through the agency of animal substances are easily discovered. The natural condition of the nose, the healthy state of the mucous membrane of the nasal fossæ, and the insensibility of the tumors, would all serve to disclose the cheat. The extraction of the foreign body itself, or its expulsion provoked by sneezing artificially produced, after the surgeon has satisfied himself that it is not held by any thread passing through the posterior nares, and fastened to one of the back teeth, will finally determine the question as to its true origin and character.

Ozæna.

§ 181. An unnatural flatness of the nose, or the presence of polypi, by blocking the nasal passages, and preventing the escape of their natural secretions, gives rise to a decomposition of the latter, which infects the expired air with a peculiar fetor. The disease from this circumstance has received the name of ozæna. It is also produced by an ulceration, sometimes syphilitic, of the mucous membrane of the nasal passages, of the velum palati, or of the maxillary sinus; or again it may spring from a morbid state of the constitution and independent of any local influences. Its rebellious character under treatment, whether of an internal or external form, always renders it a sufficient reason for rejecting a recruit, because of the discomfort, likely to be caused to others through its insupportable fœtor. When present in a soldier its probable causes should first be ascertained, and the chances of its curability, before granting a discharge.

The peculiar odor emitted by ozæna is occasionally simulated by introducing into the nasal passages, sponges impregnated with putrid animal matters, or pieces of decomposed cheese.

Certain diseases giving rise to the *nasal voice*, through division of the velum palati, its permanent paralysis, perforation of its arch, or the presence of tumors in the back part of the throat, are also a suitable cause for rejection.

SECTION XXI.

DISEASES OF THE FACIAL SINUS.

§ 182. Diseases of the frontal and maxillary sinus are similar in nature to those of the nasal passages. These cavities may be deformed, obliterated or perforated by wounds, fistulas, ulcers, or fractures with depression, or even by the introduction of foreign bodies; or they may be the seat of chronic inflammation and suppuration, of exostosis, caries, or necrosis with fistulous ulceration, often dependent upon syphilis. Polypi rarely present themselves in these parts.

Occlusion.

§ 183. Occlusion of the maxillary sinus, occasions a species of œdema of these parts.

Nearly all the foregoing diseases afford causes for rejection or discharge.

SECTION XXII.

DISEASES OF THE MAXILLARY BONES.

Affections of the Superior Maxillary Bones.

§ 184. These bones when *atrophied* or *hypertrophied*, constitute a deformity.

Congenital Fissure.

§ 185. Congenital fissure of the arch of the palate, which sometimes accompanies harelip, is a cause for rejection.

Accidental Lesions.

§ 186. The upper jaw may be the seat of severe mechanical lesions, of simple or complicated wounds, of perforations or of fractures, any of which may afford causes for rejection, according to their gravity. The same rule will apply with relation to the presence of foreign bodies, ulcerations, extensive cicatrices or deformities, consequent upon surgical operations.

Perforation of the arch of the palate, may be concealed by the application of an obturator. This portion of the mouth should therefore always be explored by the touch, as well as sight. This is a frequent seat of osteo-sarcoma and epulis.

AFFECTION OF THE INFERIOR MAXILLARY BONES.

Congenital Lesions.

§ 187. The lower jaw is a very common seat of disease. Its atrophy produces not only a painful deformity, but a defect of harmony between the rows of teeth. The same result follows its undue prominence. Either of these congenital lesions is a cause for rejection. But inasmuch as prominence of the lower jaw may be simulated by voluntary and momentary effort, it is well to make the recruit speak in order to detect the cheat.

Accidental Lesions.

§ 188. Ununited or badly-united fractures, or loss of substance of this bone, either from gun-shot wounds, or resections, are disqualifications for the military service. Other diseases are also often observed there, such as ostitis, caries, necrosis, particularly the phosphoric necrosis, bony cysts—all which generally unfit a man for military service.

Temporo-Maxillary Articulation.

§ 189. The temporo-maxillary articulation is often the seat of disqualifying diseases, such as an imperfectly reduced luxation, which impedes mastication, or a facility of luxation often of a voluntary character.

Contraction and Anchylosis.

§ 190. Contraction or closing of the jaws which may be either congenital, accidental or resulting from the influences of mercury, is a cause for rejection; anchylosis (a rare thing) is its most aggravated form.

In order to ascertain the reality of this condition, when alleged to exist, the index finger of each hand should be pushed into the hollow formed between the mastoid process and the ascending angle of the lower jaw, at the same time strongly compressing the nerves of the facial branch at their point of emergence. The pain consequent upon this operation immediately does away with the contraction, if it be voluntary and simulated.

SECTION XXIII.

DISEASES OF THE MOUTH.

§ 191. The mouth serving as it does the threefold purposes of mastication, respiration, and speech, often presents some of the greatest disqualifications for the military service. A curved spatula for depressing the tongue is very useful in its examination.

DISEASES OF THE LIPS.

Skin Diseases.

§ 192. The lips are often visited by severe skin diseases, which give cause for rejection whenever they do not promptly and evidently yield to medical treatment. The disgusting appearance presented by these affections, and their repulsiveness in the eyes of soldiers, obliged to live in common, is an additional reason for their being a disqualification. Mentagra in particular, which consists in a pustular eruption about the lips and chin, and whose duration can rarely be determined, should always cause the rejection of a recruit. This disease is sometimes feigned, but always in so gross a way as to give little trouble to the surgeon in discovering it. No directions need be given.

Hypertrophy.—Contraction.—Accidental Harelip.

§ 193. The upper lip may be hypertrophied to such a degree as to constitute a true deformity, and to impede distinctness of articulation. So also burns and ulcerations, by causing adherent cicatrices about the orifice of the mouth, may occasion its contraction to such an extent as to produce deformity, or impair the freedom of its use. A lip, from a wound, or mutilation, may be left with a form of accidental harelip, or either of them may be wanting in whole, or in part, together with some portion of the cheek; again, the upper lip may be the seat of a congenital fissure, sufficiently extensive to impede speech and even mastication, if the split be large enough to expose the teeth up to the gums.

Excessive swelling of the upper lip may be produced by the sting of an insect (e. g., bee, or wasp), or the application of some irritant, but the extent of the swelling, heat, tension, redness, and shiny appearance, renders it readily distinguishable from a chronic swelling, which latter proceeds, almost always, from a scrofulous habit.

Labial Paralysis.

§ 194. The muscles designed to move the lips and the cheeks, and supplied by the facial nerve, may be paralyzed either simply, or jointly with the orbicular muscle of the eyelids, and those giving motion to the alæ nasi. In such cases the lips are completely immovable, and unable either to seize, or to retain food, which escapes, together with the saliva, from the paralyzed side of the mouth, while certain vowels and labial consonants can scarcely be articulated. The cheek being flaccid cannot perform its office, either of mastication or deglutition. This form of paralysis, in its effects upon the competency of recruits, falls into the same class with that of the orbicular muscle of the eyelids.

Stomatitis.

§ 195. Stomatitis, or inflammation of the mouth, may arise from different causes, producing likewise different effects upon the question of qualification. As a general rule, this disorder is of trivial consequence, unless dependent upon some constitutional impairment. Thus it may be either diphtheritic, scrofulous, syphilitic, scorbutic, mercurial, ulcerous, or gangrenous. Some of these forms are manifestly of easy cure, while others require too long a treatment to tolerate the acceptance of any recruit laboring under them. *Gangrene* of the mouth, for example, always is a cause for rejection, owing to the loss of substance, the imperfect or adherent cicatrices, and the perforations or fistulas, which it generally determines.

Fetor of Breath.

§ 196. Stomatitis often occasions fetid breath. This condition arises also, frequently, from a carious state of the teeth, or some lesion of the stomach. In either case it may render a man insupportable to his companions, and thus justify his rejection, or even his discharge. When arising simply from an uncleanly state of the mouth, the cause is readily removable; and when simulated by the swallowing of fetid substances, the cheat can be easily discovered by the different nature of the odor emitted.

Diseases of the Gums.

§ 197. Shrinking of the gums, giving rise to loosening of the teeth, is always a cause for rejection.

Inflammation of the Gums (Gingivitis).

§ 198. Chronic gingivitis, ulceration, or hæmorrhage, which are easily provoked or simulated, are not causes for rejection, unless dependent upon scurvy, anæmia, &c., &c.

Scorbutic Condition.

§ 199. Irritating and corrosive substances applied to the gums may give rise to appearances, simulating those of scurvy; but it is impossible to imitate the sero-sanguinolent discharge, which flows from the gums on the least touch, the deposit of sordes upon the teeth, or their loosening, as observed in the real disease. Mercurial preparations might, to a certain extent, produce analogous effects, but the specific inflammation of the mouth always following their use, ulcerations on the edges of the tongue, and salivation, characterized by its abundance and its peculiar odor, would readily reveal the original source of the mischief.

THE TEETH AND THEIR DISEASES.

Loss of Teeth.

§ 200. Besides the office of mastication performed by the teeth, they are essential to the soldier for the purpose of tearing his cartridge, and when they cannot do this for him, he is disqualified for the military service. The soldier must have enough sound teeth to chew the food composing his rations, particularly hard bread. Admitting all other teeth to be sound, the recruit must still be rejected when he presents the following dental conditions, viz.:

1st. Loss or decay of the four incisors of the same jaw.

2d. Loss or decay of the two lateral incisors or cuspids of each jaw.

3d. Loss or caries of several incisors or cuspids in either jaw (five at least).

Where the other teeth are not in a state of soundness, the recruit should likewise be rejected. If some of the molars are wanting, the others should at least be sound together with the gums, otherwise the latter are exposed to frequent irritation, to swelling, and to recurrences of disease under the slightest exciting causes. Whenever therefore a bad state of the teeth is accompanied by softening, chronic ulceration, livid and sanguinolent swelling of the gums, or an impaired state of the constitution, the recruit must be rejected. But, on the other hand, if the teeth are, generally speaking, sound, and only disfigured by sordes, and if the constitution be good there is no cause for rejection. Among soldiers, the loss of many teeth (the cuspids always excepted) without accompanying disease of the gums, or of the constitution, does not necessarily prevent their usefulness nor justify their discharge.

Congenital Absence of Teeth.

§ 201. Congenital absence of several teeth is not a disqualification in a recruit, so long as the remainder are duly and orderly placed.

Absence of teeth may, undoubtedly, be the result of criminal design, and in such cases, it will be difficult for the surgeon always to detect the fact. Presumption in favor of natural loss will arise, whenever the remaining teeth are unsound, the gums fungous, ulcerated, &c., and the constitution enfeebled: still, an opposite condition of things does not certainly prove fraud. Finding the fangs of the teeth cut off on a level with the alveolar process, is not, as has been generally supposed, a proof of deception, because certain forms of decay or accidents may have occasioned it.

Again, loss of teeth may be concealed by the introduction of artificial ones; to guard against which, a critical examination of the mouth should always be made.

Dental Anomalies.

§ 202. Anomalies of the teeth must be duly considered, and investigated, under the light of their possible influence as exciting causes of disease of the maxillary bones. These diseases have already been alluded to.

Supernumerary Teeth.

§ 203. Supernumerary teeth, although occasioning no discomfort, may yet produce a sufficient deformity to require the rejection of a recruit.

Deviation and Fistulas.

§ 204. Deviation of the teeth, unless in the most exceptional instances, cannot be considered as a disqualification.

So with dental fistulas, which are cured by the extraction of the diseased tooth.

Diseases of the Tongue.

§ 205. The tongue being an organ of indispensable use in the processes of mastication, deglutition, or articulation, any serious lesion of it must therefore be a disqualification for the military service.

Prolapsus.—Congenital Division.—Hypertrophy.

§ 206. Prolapsus of the tongue, which is a rare congenital affection, is productive of salivation, and always a cause for rejection. The same is the case with *bifid* tongue, or a hypertrophied state of that organ, consequent upon inflammation, and exposing its subject to the danger of asphyxia.

Mechanical Lesions.

§ 207. Various mechanical lesions, such as wounds arising from bites, accidents, or convulsions, may give occasion for rejection, according to their extent or original cause.

Partial Loss.

§ 208. The same rule will follow in partial loss of the tongue, which, if inconsiderable and traumatic, is not a disqualification for military service.

Retraction.

§ 209. Retraction of the tongue, which may be either spasmodic, progressive, primitive, or consecutive, is not a disqualification in itself. The original cause and the gravity of the lesion, must in each case determine the question.

Abnormal Adhesions.

§ 210. The mobility of the tongue, being an indispensable condition for the performance of its functions, any thing interfering with it in the nature of abnormal adhesions, consequent upon acute or ulcerative inflammation, or extensive lesions, forms evidently a disqualification for the military service. But, inasmuch as many of these deformities readily yield to surgical treatment, it does not follow that their presence among soldiers, necessarily justifies a discharge, and not until art has failed in her resources, or nature reproduces the deformity with resistless obstinacy, should this be granted.

Stammering.

§ 211. Stammering, from whatever cause arising, is an absolute disqualification for the military service; not only because it prevents *challenging*, or giving the countersign, but, because it acts as an insuperable bar to the promotion of men, by disabling them from giving the word of command. Tenotomy, which was formerly practised in such cases, is now entirely abandoned.

From the fact that, most frequently, the mouth exhibits no alterations in structure, by which to explain the cause of this disorder, stammering is among those disabilities most apt to be feigned. The duty of the surgeon in such cases is, by examining all their probabilities, and comparing them with public report, to determine whether the actual state of things is a natural, or a counterfeit, or exaggerated one.

Dumbness.

§ 212. Dumbness, which as we have before stated, is often congenital, and the result of deafness, may also be accidental, symptomatic of cerebral disease, or the result of a wound, atrophy, hypertrophy, or paralysis of the tongue. Of all the foregoing causes, the last only can be feigned. In inquiring into the possible causes of this, it is necessary to ascertain whether any disease of the brain has previously existed, or if any blow or wound of the head has ever been received. When there is real paralysis, the tongue is thin, emaciated, and, as it were, rolled together, and the same cause which prevents articulation, prevents it also from being thrust out; whence the saying, that every dumb man, not born deaf, who can thrust his tongue out, and move it, is an impostor.

Diseases of the Velum Palati.

§ 213. Diseases of the *velum palati* are of important consideration, on account of their influence upon respiration, deglutition, and phonation.

Congenital Absence.—Division.—Loss of Substance.

§ 214. Congenital absence of the velum palati, whether total or partial, is rare. It always justifies rejection.

Its congenital or acquired fissures, losses of substance consequent upon wounds or ulcerations, tumors which may have their seat there, adhesions following inflamma tions or operations, and which are liable to close the posterior opening of the nasal passages, are all causes for rejection or discharge, whenever these lesions, combined with double and congenital division of the upper lip, affect the voice, and interfere with deglutition. It is more particularly so, when the arch of the palate shares this deformity in common with the velum.

Diphtheritic Paralysis.

§ 215. Diphtheritic paralysis, which is generally relieved by time, and without treatment, can only in extraordinary cases, justify rejection.

Diseases of the Uvula.

§ 216. Elongation of the uvula from relaxation of its tissue, œdema, or hypertrophy, produces a series of discomforts, such as incessant tickling, desire to swallow, at times a slight cough, or even frequent vomiting. As this condition is not a serious one, a slight surgical operation being sufficient to relieve the patient, it furnishes no cause for rejection, unless the uvula were not simply hypertrophied, but also the seat of cancerous degeneration. The question of discharge is still less to be considered.

Diseases of the Salivary Glands.

§ 217. The saliva being essential to digestion, the integrity of the glands concerned in its elaboration, becomes, therefore, an all-important prerequisite to health.

These glands are subject to alterations, bearing a great analogy to those of the lachrymal apparatus. The parotid, submaxillary, and sublingual, may be enlarged or degenerated; their secretions may escape involuntarily from the mouth, or be retained in the excretory ducts, occasioning a tumor, or even escape by a fistulous opening.

Chronic Enlargements.—Degeneration.

§ 218. Chronic enlargements, hypertrophy, or degeneration of the foregoing glands, which are diseases of rather an uncommon character, refractory under treatment, and dependent upon disordered constitutional habit, belong more properly among diseases of the neck, under which head we shall accordingly notice them. The same is the case with hypertrophy of the submaxillary and sublingual glands, often confounded with submaxillary adenitis.

Involuntary flow of Saliva.

§ 219. Involuntary flow of saliva being always a secondary affection, its original cause is the proper subject of inquiry for the surgeon, for it may arise from loss of substance of the lower lip, paralysis, syphilis, &c., &c. This affection is easily feigned.

Ranula.

§ 220. The most common salivary tumor is ranula, which develops itself under the tongue, and impedes more or less its motion. It is frequently the result of salivary calculi, and always affords a cause for rejection, and often for discharge, because of its tendency to recur even after having been subjected to surgical treatment.

Salivary Fistulas.

§ 221. Salivary fistulas, usually the result of wounds, are difficult of cure, and always afford a cause for rejection, and often for discharge.

Atrophy and Hypertrophy of the Tonsils.

§ 222. Absence or atrophy of the tonsils, which is generally more apparent than real, is not a cause for rejection.

Chronic enlargement or hypertrophy of these glands, consequent upon repeated inflammation, is not a cause for rejection, until they have become so large, as sensibly to impede deglutition, hearing, phonation, or respiration.

Discharges should rarely be granted for this cause, since simple excision of the tonsils will most generally produce a radical cure of the disorder.

SECTION XXIV.

DISEASES OF THE NECK.

Deformities.

§ 223. Atrophy or congenital narrowness, or, on the other hand, excessive development of the neck out of all proportion to the head, or thorax, are at times observed, and may thus constitute a cause for rejection.

Ulcers, Cicatrices, and Scrofulous Enlargements.

§ 224. It is in the region of the neck that a scrofulous habit of body characterizes itself most strongly. Chronic enlargement of the cervical and submaxillary ganglia, abscesses, ulcers, and the cicatrices which they leave, all indicate a diseased constitution, and an unfitness to perform the duties of a soldier. Any of the lymphatic ganglia of the neck, may be the seat of scrofulous enlargement, but the submaxillary are generally points of election.

Scrofulous ulcerations of the neck, voluminous or multiple tumors of a similar nature, and the cicatrices resulting from their suppuration, when extensive and imperfect, are always causes for rejection. As to discharges, they should be granted only when the disease has successfully resisted medical treatment, or produced changes in the body, incompatible with the performance of a soldier's duties.

Glandular Tumors.

§ 225. Glandular tumors, which are of frequent occurrence in the army, and present themselves under a variety of aspects, being generally known as the *cervical adenitis of soldiers*, are, when large, and of a chronic character, causes both for rejection and discharge. Care must be taken not to confound these tumors with enlargement of the post-cervical glands, symptomatic of secondary syphilis.

Varieties of Tumors.

§ 226. Aside from the diseases common to all parts of the surface of the body, various tumors may specially manifest themselves in the region of the neck; such as in front and below, enlargement of the thoracic or subclavian glands, and aneurism of the arch of the aorta; in front and above, ranula and bursal enlargement; on the sides, large parotid tumors, and disease of the cervical vertebræ. These different manifestations of disease plainly indicate to the surgeon the judgment he should pronounce.

Goitre.

§ 227. The term *goitre* is applied to nearly all the tumors which develop themselves in the thyroid gland. Chronic hypertrophy of this gland, whether partial or complete, parenchymatous or cystic, simple or complicated, constitutes a cause for rejection. In soldiers, no discharge is justifiable until the disease has passed into the chronic state.

An attempt to feign goitre by the introduction of air into the cellular tissue would have no chance of success.

But this disease, when slight and incipient, may be concealed. On which account, the thyroid region should always be closely scrutinized, and whenever the goitrous tumor is perceived, whatever may be its size, the party should be rejected.

Torticollis.

§ 228. The inclination of the head towards one shoulder, with deviation of the face towards the opposite side, constitutes torticollis, or wry neck. This disease may arise from a variety of causes, viz.:

1st. It may be congenital, or may have supervened in early childhood, as a result of nervous disorders.

2d. Bridled cicatrices may cause it.

3d. It sometimes arises from contractions or accidental paralyses of the sterno-mastoid muscles; or,

4th. It arises from certain spasmodic affections of the muscular system, such as nervous contractions.

Torticollis may originate in either the cutaneous, fibrous, muscular, and tendinous tissue, or in the cervical vertebræ.

First form.—When the inclination of the head is congenital, it is always accompanied by a modification in the bony structure of the face, the skull, and the neck. If the disease dates from childhood, this modification instead of being contemporaneous with, or a cause of, the inclination, is consecutive to it, and progressively increased by the growth of the subject. This form of torticollis constitutes an absolute disqualification.

One of the constant and most striking effects of this deformity, is the inequality produced in the two sides of the face—on the one hand from atrophy of the side, corresponding to the inclination, and which atrophy extends to the bony structure, as well as to the soft tissues, and on the other hand, dragging down of the same parts in the direction of the contraction. The cervical portion of the spine inclines laterally upon the first dorsal vertebra, in an opposite direction from the inclination of the head, whence it follows that on this latter side the supra-scapular space attains a greater length than on the opposite side. The mastoid process, corresponding with the infirmity, is sometimes longer than that of the other side; and an analogous difference is at times remarked in the prominence and curve of the clavicles. Finally, the motions of the head, although limited and modified, are not suspended.

Second form.—The presence of *cicatrices* explain sufficiently the mechanism of this variety of torticollis to leave no doubt as to the decision proper in relation to rejection or discharge.

Third form.—Contraction or retraction of one or several of the muscles which bend the head upon the body, and particularly of the sterno-mastoideus, whether resulting from convulsive rigidity, paralysis, or defective antagonism of opposing muscles, occasions an abnormal inclination, to which also the name of torticollis has been given. The *acute* form, which is easily curable, does not incapacitate for the duties of a soldier; it can be recognized by the sharp pain occasioned by any attempt at straightening the head, but chiefly by the absence of the characteristic signs of long standing torticollis, or that which springs from muscular retraction.

Fourth form.—When torticollis springs from paralysis, it is usually the sterno-cleido-mastoideus which suffers. In such case, the head leans towards the healthy side, while the face looks towards the affected side. This is the opposite of what is observed in torticollis from contraction. The head can be easily, and without pain, returned to its natural position, but as soon as its support is removed, it resumes its faulty position. This disease is a cause for rejection, but not of discharge, until the paralysis has shown itself incurable.

It is evident, therefore, that congenital torticollis cannot be feigned, on account of the characteristic structural changes which, in various degrees, ever accompany it.

When torticollis springs from muscular contraction, the affected muscle towards which the head leans, forms beneath the skin a kind of stretched cord, prominent, resisting pressure, which opposes straightening by an equal and passive action, and which, neither distracting the attention of the party, nor force, unless excessive, can overcome.

In torticollis from paralysis, the healthy muscle which draws the head to its own side, shows neither extraordinary rigidity, nor hardness; but the opposite muscle, being deprived of activity, is soft, flaccid, inert, and, as it were, lost in the surrounding soft parts, and whatever may be the motions of straightening or rotation imparted to the head, it shows no signs of contraction. These symptomatic details, when well understood, will always enable the surgeon to distinguish the real disease, since simulators could hardly imitate them with sufficient accuracy to deceive him.

From whatever source arising, torticollis always constitutes a cause for rejection. Discharges should also be granted in those cases arising from cicatrices or traumatic lesions, and where art is ineffectual to relieve them.

The *organs of the voice* are so essential also to the soldier, that every obstacle to speech is a disqualification for the military service.

SECTION XXV.

DISEASES OF THE LARYNX AND TRACHEA.

Lesions.

§ 229. Both the larynx and trachea may be the seat of traumatic lesions, such as wounds, ulcers, fistulas, followed by adherent cicatrices, resulting either from wounds or tracheotomy; the thyroid cartilage may be fractured, or foreign bodies, though rarely, may lodge themselves in these organs.

These lesions are all causes for rejection, but justify a discharge, only when likely to be followed by serious complications.

Laryngitis.

§ 230. Acute laryngitis constitutes a disqualification only in serious cases, whose complexion is to be judged by the surgeon. The *pseudo*-membranous form presents danger enough always to justify rejection.

Chronic Diseases.

§ 231. Chronic affections of the larynx, although at times obscure in their local symptoms, yet always produce, when severe, a condition of system, which is eminently suggestive to the observer. The relations which ordinarily exist between chronic lesions of the larynx and those of the lungs, should always cause the rejection of parties suffering under the former. These structural changes present themselves especially under the form of ulcerations of the larynx, and necrosis of its cartilages, or laryngeal phthisis, narrowing of the larynx resulting sometimes from laryngeo-tracheotomy, the presence of tumors, or of polypi.

These lesions often occasion an alteration of, and even a complete loss of voice (*aphonia*), sufficient in itself to disqualify a person for military service.

Aphonia.

§ 232. Permanent aphonia sometimes exists without any appreciable material lesion, although the laryngoscope may have been employed with a view to diminish the number of such obscure cases.

It constitutes even then a cause for rejection; but when presenting itself among soldiers it is well to try the efficacy of treatment before granting a discharge. In order to ascertain the reality of this affection, the surgeon must proceed by induction, and on the same principles laid down for cases of amaurosis and deafness. Aphonia is, in fact, at times feigned, and simulators have exhibited a degree of pertinacity under examination, sufficient to thwart for a long while, the tests to which they were subjected.

Feigned aphonia is generally recognized by the absence of sibilant sounds, of efforts at expiration, and of the swelling of the jugular veins, as well as of those of the anterior portion of the neck. In doubtful cases after a critical examination of the neck, the pharynx, and the test with sternutatories, or coughing produced by breathing sulphurous acid, or chlorine, nothing remains but to try harsh and unexpected impressions; a cry emitted, or a word spoken aloud, in such cases, suffices to expose the cheat.

SECTION XXVI.

DISEASES OF THE PHARYNX.

§ 233. Diseases of the pharynx and œsophagus, by interfering with deglutition, may occasion serious impairment of the function of nutrition, and produce, when prolonged, a marked emaciation, profound debility, and general prostration.

Anomalies of the Pharynx.

§ 234. Anomalies of the pharynx, although rare, may occasionally present themselves. They would not afford a cause for rejection, unless there was sensible deformity, or something in the nature of a diverticulum (*cul-de-sac*), as has been sometimes observed.

Traumatic Lesions.

§ 235. Traumatic lesions of the pharynx, resulting from transverse, sub, or supra-hyoideal wounds, and occasioned by attempts at homicide, or suicide, even when fully cicatrized, require that the party should be either rejected or discharged.

Foreign Bodies.

§ 236. Foreign bodies which find their way into the

walls of the pharynx, such as fragments of bones, or small projectiles, are causes for rejection or discharge, according to the difficulty of their extraction, or the consequences produced by their presence. Foreign bodies, when swallowed, tend to pass from the pharynx into the stomach, thence to lose themselves in the bowels, or to make their way out of the body through different organs.

Pharyngitis.

§ 237. Inflammation of the pharynx becomes a cause for rejection, only by reason of its serious results and of their complications.

Diphtheria.

§ 238. Diphtheria, extending beyond the pharynx, is ever a disqualification in a recruit, and gangrenous angina equally so.

Retro-Pharyngeal Abscess.

§ 239. Abscesses formed behind the pharynx, do not generally arise from its inflammation, however severe this may be, but from more profound lesions, and particularly, from caries of the upper cervical vertebræ. They constitute retro-pharyngeal abscess, which is symptomatic of disease of a joint, and requires either the rejection, or discharge of its subject.

Ulcers.

§ 240. Ulcers of the pharynx, or of the isthmus faucium, most generally of syphilitic origin, are not a cause for rejection, unless they extend deeply and involve neighboring parts; such, for example, as the arch or the pillars of the palate.

SECTION XXVII.

DISEASES OF THE ŒSOPHAGUS.

Malformation.—Foreign Bodies.

§ 241. The œsophagus may be the seat of various malformations, which it is here needless to enumerate. Among mechanical lesions, it is only necessary to cite foreign bodies, whose presence may afford cause for rejection. To justify a discharge, it would be necessary that the impossibility of either withdrawing them, or forcing them down, had been shown.

Dysphagia.

§ 242. The subject of dysphagia presents itself, not only under the aspect of traumatic lesions, but also with relation to various diseases, such as spasmodic stricture, either a purely nervous disease, or symptomatic of inflammation, stricture, partial dilatation, paralysis, softening (analogous to that of the intestine), ulcerations, cancer, &c. These diseases, although rarely encountered by examining surgeons, are frequently seen in hospitals, and ever afford a cause for discharge.

Dysphagia, from whatever cause arising, is always accompanied by an impairment of the general health. An examination of the bodily condition must always be made, whenever any suspicions of the reality of this affection arise.

Paralysis.

§ 243. Paralysis of the pharynx and of the œsophagus, is an affection rarely occurring, except as a symptom of serious nervous disease, and occasioning as a consequence, whenever prolonged, marked emaciation, profound debility and general prostration,—results, whose absence would set at defiance all such attempts at feigning as contortions during deglutition, efforts to vomit, to cough, to sneeze, by means of which an obstacle would be put to the entrance of food or drink into the pharynx, or those nervous spasms causing solid or fluid substances to be rejected through the nostrils, during deglutition. It is needless to remark that this affection is always a cause for rejection or for discharge, when incurable.

Coarctation, (Stricture).

§ 244. Difficulty of swallowing may arise from stricture of the œsophagus, without any appreciable external sign of this alteration. It may be discovered, however, by introducing into the œsophagus, a gum elastic sound. A urethral catheter of largest size, provided with a stylet, and slightly curved, will answer for this purpose.

By the obstacle encountered, and the sense of friction transmitted, it is easy to establish the existence, the situation, and the degree of contraction, of the stricture. This latter always affords a cause for rejection. A discharge should, likewise, always be granted, even though, by the employment of dilating instruments, a cure seems to have been obtained; because, in the first place, such a cure is never complete, and secondly, because the disease has a tendency to return in a more aggravated form under the influence of army diet, however good it may otherwise be. Feigning can be discovered by practising catheterism.

SECTION XXVIII.

DISEASES OF THE CERVICAL VERTEBRÆ.

Articular Torticollis.—Cervical Sprain.

§ 245. Diseases of the cervical vertebræ, require a critical examination, either by pressure with the fingers in the posterior region of the neck, or by exploring the posterior fauces, and particularly the pharynx. Touch will also enable us to discover certain congenital deformities or deviations of the bony structure of those parts (articular torticollis), or among anatomical lesions, cervical sprain, recent or of long standing, varying according to the degree of pain, the extent of deviation, and the immobility of the vertebræ, whose ligaments had suffered distension or partial rupture. The peculiar and persistent attitude of the head, well known to surgeons, is a pathognomonic sign of the disease, in its early stage. These diseases are always a cause for rejection. Feigned cervical sprain is of too easy discovery to require any special notice. The means to be employed by the surgeon in ascertaining its reality, require prudence and careful manipulation.

Fracture.

§ 246. Fracture or incomplete luxation of the cervical vertebræ, occasioning more serious effects than sprains, and creating danger of compression of the cord, leave no room for doubt as to the decision which should be made.

Other Diseases.

§ 247. Diseases of the *cervical vertebræ*, or their articulations, impairing permanently, or seriously, the motions of the neck, whether arising from wounds, rheumatism, or scrofula, are a cause for rejection.

There is a serious condition sometimes resulting from one of the foregoing, which must not be overlooked in this connection. It is a form of white swelling, occipito-vertebral caries, which may suddenly complicate itself with spontaneous or symptomatic luxation, and thus produce instant death. Hence the necessity of carefully examining every one, presenting any appearance of this disease. Feigning of this would be almost impossible, before any practised surgeon.

SECTION XXIX.

DISEASES OF THE CHEST AND BACK.

General Considerations.

§ 248. The chest contains the principal organs of respiration, and of circulation, whose continuous and regular play is essentially necessary for the maintenance of life or health. It also acts as a point of support in the performance of many movements, and particularly of extraordinary efforts. And lastly, in a military point of view, it directly supports the hardest and heaviest portions of the equipment, such as the knapsack and other accoutrements. Under these various aspects, the condition of the chest in recruits should receive the most attentive examination. An external examination of the chest, enables us to appreciate its general conformation, and the different lesions which may exist upon its exterior walls, such as wounds, ulcers, scars, tumors, &c., &c. Mensuration of the chest with a tape measure, will also afford valuable indications touching the dimensions of this cavity, in its relations to the size of the body, as well as to the volume of the important organs within.

Internal examination by means of auscultation* and percussion, reveals the principal diseases of the respiratory organs, and of the heart. Diseases of the chest having a melancholy frequency in the army, make it incumbent upon examining surgeons, to carefully scrutinize all recruits in this particular, with relation to latent predispositions.

The *form* of the chest may disclose through its various peculiarities, the state of the contained organs, and thus acquire great importance in every examination of a recruit. In a well-built man, the thorax is broad and prominently convex; the ribs are long and symmetrically arched; the shoulder-blades not prominent, and well covered by the muscles which move them and fill their cavities. In this portion of the trunk, many causes for rejection may be found.

DISEASES OF THE THORAX.

Deformities.

§ 249. Congenital deformities of the chest have their origin more particularly in its bony walls, but first of all, in the spinal column, whose deviations and curvatures

* It is a good plan, in auscultating a party, to place him with his back against a wooden door or partition. The greater resonance of the pectoral sounds obtained by this process, will surprise those who have never before availed themselves of this simple acoustic medium.

ordinarily produce relative deformities of the ribs and sternum. Rachitis is, moreover, a complex disease, and not restrained to the vertebral column alone, however great may be its deviations. Deformities of the chest may be enumerated as follows, viz.:

Prominence of the thorax, in the shape of a ship's kee (pigeon-breast). The cartilages of the ribs being straight, instead of prolonging the arched curve of the ribs.

Depression, at times considerable, of the lower portion of the sternum, and the ensiform cartilage, with inversion or eversion of it.

Extreme narrowness of the sterno-costal walls, best proved by mensuration.

Every one whose chest does not measure thirty-one and a half inches in circumference, should be rejected, as unfit for military service; for rarely are such chests large or strong enough to enable the contained viscera to perform their functions without hindrance, and in particular, for the lungs to have full play.

Among other causes for rejection may be noted, curvatures of different kinds, partial deviation of the ribs and sternum, exaggerated mobility of the floating ribs, defective ossification of some portions of the sternum, which with a bifid state of this bone, are both of rare occurrence.

Wounds.

§ 250. Wounds of the chest may occasion consequences which often, but not invariably, afford causes for rejection or discharge.

Foreign Bodies.

§ 251. Foreign bodies of various kinds, such as projectiles and splinters, may be lodged in the walls of the chest, and again extracted, or may penetrate its cavity. No general rule can be laid down touching the importance of such lesions. An attentive examination of each case is necessary to enable the surgeon to arrive at a correct decision.

Lesions of the Lungs.

§ 252. Contusions, lacerations, wounds, or hernia of the lungs, generally constitute serious lesions. The last named may be produced by other causes than a penetrating wound—may be congenital, or arise from an effort of coughing. Hernia of the lung, through the cicatrix of a wound, exhibits itself in the form of a soft, circumscribed tumor, which rises and falls with the respiratory movements. It is easily reducible, and then exposes the cavity into which the pulmonary parenchyma has escaped, to view, through the cicatrix. Auscultation reveals the presence of air in the cells of the tumor.

Traumatic Emphysema.

§ 253. Traumatic emphysema of the lung—pneumonia, and traumatic pleuritis—traumatic effusions, whether sanguineous, serous, or purulent, into the pleura or pericardium, paracentesis thoracis, and its consequences—all these surgical affections afford a cause for rejection, but not always for discharge.

SECTION XXX.

DISEASES OF THE RIBS AND STERNUM.

Mechanical Lesions.

§ 254. The structure of the solid framework of the chest composed of bones and cartilages, imparts to this portion of the trunk an elasticity, which enables it to resist very considerable violence. Nevertheless, all the lesions peculiar to its several tissues, may at times be observed: such as depression of the ribs, fracture of these bones, or of their cartilages, when non-consolidated or imperfectly consolidated. This form of fracture is always a cause for rejection, but its cure is so easy, whenever it is free from complications, that these alone can authorize the granting of a discharge.

Fracture of the sternum, and sterno-costal luxation, are rare; still, the foregoing rules will apply to them also. Defective ossification of this bone, or an undue mobility of its different segments, constitute a disqualification for military service. The same rule should obtain where the cartilage of one or more ribs is wanting.

Sterno-costal Ostitis.

§ 255. Ostitis and exostosis, caries and necrosis, and osteo-sarcoma of the ribs, or of the sternum, are of frequent occurrence in the army, and entail the consequences, already enumerated, as belonging to such diseases. Whatever may be the results of resecting one of these bones, they, still, always afford a cause for rejection and frequently for discharge.

SECTION XXXI.

DISEASES OF THE CLAVICLE AND OF THE CLAVICULAR REGION.

Aneurism of the Subclavian Artery.

§ 256. The clavicular region may be the seat of various tumors, of which, one in particular—aneurism of the subclavian—exhibits a special character, and pro duces the consequence already stated of such diseases.

Deformity of the Clavicle.

§ 257. The clavicle may suffer an arrest of development, or may have been subjected to irregular or faulty curvature, either through organic causes, or the results of non, or badly united, fractures; in this latter case, it often exhibits a voluminous callus, which, with the foregoing lesions, affords a cause for rejection, but not necessarily for discharge. Unreduced luxations are an absolute disqualification for military service.

SECTION XXXII.

DISEASES OF THE MAMMÆ.

Hypertrophy.

§ 258. Diseases of the mammary gland are sufficiently frequent to merit the attention of the surgeon. Hypertrophy of this gland, coincident or not, with atrophy ot the testicle, is sometimes noticed. This abnormal development constitutes, when well marked, a cause for rejection, and sometimes even for discharge.

Mammitis.

§ 259. Inflammation of the mammary gland is not infrequent among young soldiers. It may occasion hypertrophy, or induration, and justify a discharge.

Phlegmonous Tumor.

§ 260. Phlegmonous tumors, developed within the tissue of this gland, may be extensive enough to justify the discharge of a party, but rarely his rejection. These tumors are sometimes the result of tattooing, a pernicious practice of common adoption in the army.

SECTION XXXIII.

DISEASES OF THE THORACIC ORGANS.

§ 261. The large number of young soldiers who succumb to pulmonary diseases in military hospitals, particularly to phthisis, owing to the careless manner in which they have been allowed to pass before Boards of Enrolment, should impart additional watchfulness to surgeons when examining them.

Deformity of the Thorax, from Internal Causes.

§ 262. Faulty conformations of the thorax, resulting from internal diseases, which interrupt either respiration or circulation, or prevent the bearing of arms, are absolute causes for rejection or discharge. Thus, for example, old pulmonary emphysema, imparts to the chest a bulging globular form; in its early stages, however, this disease produces only partial bulging in the subclavian and sterno-mammary regions. Pleuritic effusions often reveal themselves by analogous bulgings of the posterior walls of the thorax. Resorption of these effusions is, on the other hand, frequently followed by retraction of one of the sides of the chest.

Bronchitis and Chronic Pneumonia.

§ 263. Bronchitis and chronic pneumonia, accompanied by wasting, always justify either rejection or discharge.

Pulmonary Emphysema.

§ 264. Pulmonary emphysema necessarily requires rejection. This disease, of frequent occurrence in the army, justifies a discharge only when sufficiently extensive to produce spasms of suffocation.

Phthisis.

§ 265. Threatened consumption and, for still stronger reasons, the fully developed disease, in any stage, well recognized, are disqualifications for military service. This sad predisposition reveals itself through features that are unmistakable to the physician. The chest is narrow, and only slightly muscular around its superior periphery; the shoulder-blades are prominent and detached; the neck is long; the countenance pale or flushed about the cheek-bones; the voice husky, speech hurried, and frequently interrupted by the necessity of breathing; the skin is fine and transparent, or presents a sallow look, and an unnatural dryness; the limbs are emaciated, and covered by lean and flaccid muscles.

In addition to the impressions produced by these *indicia*, judgment must be further enlightened by recourse to percussion, auscultation, and mensuration. Too many proofs cannot be accumulated, on a subject involving such important consequences. Unusual dulness over any part of the chest; absence or modification of the respiratory murmur; inordinate development, or retraction of either side of this cavity, will leave no doubt as to the state of the lungs, or the pleura, and the necessity for a rejection or discharge of the individual.

We must not expect to find all these symptoms united in any one person. The presence of a few characteristic ones should suffice to justify a rejection whenever they establish, not only the confirmed disease, but even a strong predisposition to it.

The fingers and the ear serve for immediate percussion and auscultation. Mensuration should be effected by a tape measure, as described in section 8; but in order to render this element of diagnosis valuable, it is indispensable for the surgeon to bear in mind the different dimensions and relative proportions of a well-formed chest. See section 248.

An important sign, and one too, which, in the midst of the difficulties surrounding percussion and auscultation, can always be determined, is the comparison between the number of respirations and pulsations. The normal standard in adults is about twenty respirations to seventy-two pulsations per minute, or as $3 \div 1$ —.

At a more advanced stage of the disease, uncertainty is impossible, so highly accentuated are all the morbid phenomena.

Sometimes recruits feign weakness of chest by rounding the back, bringing their shoulders forward, and presenting the sternum, apparently depressed; they also affect a dry, frequent cough, and reply to questions with a hurried breath. But it is only necessary to straighten the individual, and to throw back his shoulders, to discover the good development of the thorax; while at the same time the color and elasticity of the integuments, and the volume and firmness of the muscles, will all conspire to expose the cheat. The presence or absence of physical signs will determine the question.

Hæmoptysis.

§ 266. Hæmoptysis, as a symptom of pulmonary disease, is always a cause for rejection. It is also a cause for discharge, when it returns frequently, is accompanied by a persistent cough and marked emaciation, with or without the other physical signs of tuberculosis.

A soldier attacked for the first time by hæmoptysis should be subjected to close observation, for this form of hæmorrhage is often observed to be followed by a rapid development of phthisis, not alone among delicate persons disposed to scrofula, or whose chests are badly formed, but also—and this point cannot be too much dwelt upon—in apparently strong persons having a dark skin, black hair, and a well-developed muscular system.

In rarer cases, hæmoptysis is a symptom of heart disease, particularly of hypertrophy. A thorough and differential examination of the heart and lungs will enable us to establish this diagnostic point. At all events, by reason of its being the result of cardiac lesion, hæmoptysis is not the less serious, and should entail similar consequences to any other symptom of phthisis.

In order to feign it, some persons prick the finger, forearm, or any other part of the body accessible to the lips, and by suction, fill the mouth with blood, which they void immediately after having feigned a spasm of coughing. Others prick the gums and pharynx,—while some conceal under the tongue or the hollow between the teeth and cheeks, Armenian bole, or a sponge saturated with blood, from which they express variable quantities, and thus redden the saliva. The cheat is easily discovered by passing the fingers through the mouth, and rinsing it out with acidulated water. Moreover, the blood of hæmoptysis is distinguishable by its bright and frothy character; at the termination of the attack it mingles itself with and tinges the bronchial secretions of a more or less deep color, and finally, the real attack always leaves a pallor and prostration, which cannot be simulated any more than the anxious expression, which ever marks the face of the real sufferer.

Pleuritic Effusions.

§ 267. Pleuritic effusions are always a cause for rejection. They do not, however, justify a discharge, until they have resisted all treatment or produced constitutional alterations. Contraction and impaired mobility of one side of the chest, resulting from pleurisy, constitutes a cause for rejection.

Organic Lesions of the Heart.

§ 268. In common with organic lesions of the lungs, those of the heart and large blood-vessels are of difficult detection in their incipient stage. Yet the obstacles they present to the discharge of a soldier's duties, through the rapid development they undergo under the efforts incidental to military life, and the dangers they occasion in their subjects, render it of great importance that all such persons should be kept out of the army.

No means of exploration should be omitted. Recourse must be had to palpation, in order to discover the frequency, force, extent, and rhythm of the motions of the heart, and the prominence or bulging of the thorax; to auscultation, for indications of the nature and intensity of abnormal sounds; and to mensuration and percussion, which disclose increase in volume and limits of size. At the same time it will be necessary to search out, and to analyze attentively, the disturbances which these lesions may excite in the play of other organs; such as shortness of breath. Slowness or acceleration, or disturbance of the circulation, will reveal themselves through dyspnœa, often one of the first symptoms of heart disease; by the feebleness, force, irregularity, or intermission of the pulse; by the red or livid injection of the capillaries, particularly of the face, and by the distension or pulsation of the jugular veins, etc.

Besides the signs by which to distinguish dilatation of the heart, and of its sac when distended by dropsy—that is to say, besides the extension of precordial dulness, which normally does not cover more than two and a-half square inches,—the other phenomena, viewed by themselves, are far from furnishing precise or irrefragable indications. This statement applies to palpitations, to abnormal sounds, when they are slight and ephemeral, to variations of the pulse, coloration of the countenance, and the other already recited symptoms of cardiac lesion.

In such perplexing cases as these, it is only by the resemblance and the harmony of general and local symptoms, that the physician can arrive at any certain conclusions. His attention should, above all, be fixed upon the sounds of the heart, upon the relation between the strength of the pulse and the ventricular impulsions, upon the power of these, and finally upon the extent of the region occupied by the organ itself. If any uncertainty still remains, he may clear up all doubts by questioning the party upon his subjective observations of his own condition, in connection with mode of sleeping, violent exercise, and emotional excitement, &c., &c.

Displacement of the Heart.—Transposition.

§ 269. The heart may be displaced, or even totally transposed. This latter condition, which is manifestly congenital, is rare yet occasions no disorder of function; circulation and respiration going on as well with the heart on the right, as on the left side. But the same is not the case when this organ is displaced by a hepatized, or emphysematous lung, a pleuritic effusion, or the development of a morbid growth, or tumor. The simple announcement of these serious conditions suffices to indicate the opinion which the surgeon should form of their consequences.

Endocarditis.—Pericarditis.

§ 270. Acute inflammation of the heart (endocarditis), or of its sac (pericarditis), is always a cause for rejection, and often for discharge, on account of the structural alterations which it induces. Hydro-pericardium is always a cause for rejection or discharge.

Hypertrophy.

§ 271. Hypertrophy of the heart is an absolute disqualification in a recruit, and also requires the discharge of a soldier, when ordinary means of treatment have proved unavailing.

During an examination the recruit is generally excited, and the motions of the heart increased, so as to mislead one into the belief that hypertrophy is present. It may not therefore be out of place to repeat some of the physiological and pathological details, applicable to a diagnosis of this disease. In health, the intercostal muscles situated between the *fifth* and *sixth* ribs, are raised by the apex of the heart during systole, over an extent of from half an inch to one inch. In hypertrophy, these movements are much more extensive, and may include several ribs and intercostal spaces. Precordial dulness, which, in a normal state, occupies a space of two square inches, may extend itself over one of four.

Adhesion of the Pericardium.

§ 272. Friction murmur of the pericardium, indicating an altered condition of the surface of this membrane, should always cause rejection, whenever recognizable by auscultation. It should also occasion the discharge of a soldier, if accompanied by disturbances in the heart's action, and irregularity or intermission of the pulse.

Narrowing, or Insufficiency of Valves.

§ 273. Valvular sounds ordinarily announce serious lesions; rough sounds, accompany contractions of the auricular-ventricular orifices; soft ones, valvular insufficiency.

Lesions of Cardiac Orifices.—Dilatation, with Thinning.

§ 274. Purring murmurs reveal a lesion of the cardiac

orifices. Increase of precordial dulness, accompanied by feebleness of the heart's contractions and without strong impact of this organ against, nor raising of the intercostal muscles, indicates dilatation with thinning of its walls. The foregoing different conditions, as also the succeeding ones, necessarily require the rejection, or discharge of a party.

Cyanosis.

§ 275. Cyanosis, which is often an indication of the persistence of the foramen ovale, is, when congenital, beyond the reach of art.

Facial cyanosis may be produced by the application of a ligature about the base of the neck, and hidden among the folds of the skin. But in such cases there is injection and not true cyanosis, and the cheat is too clumsy to require any further notice.

Lesions of the Thoracic Aorta.

§ 276. Diagnosis of lesions of the thoracic aorta, is in most cases obscure. Yet aneurism may be suspected from the whistling of the voice, flatness of sound, on percussion over the middle and superior portions of the sternum, by the feebleness and irregularity of the pulse, and its inequality between one arm and the other. All these are *indicia* of a tumor, compressing arterial trunks, or their branches. It may also be recognized by a thrilling, or purring tremor, felt by the hand when applied to the sternum, and particularly by the simple pulsations, accompanied by a bellows murmur heard in the track of the artery. When the aneurism is situated in the ascending aorta, the pulsations are detected beneath the sternum and the cartilages of the ribs, with a distinctness corresponding to the volume of the tumor. They differ from the first sound of the heart by a greater intensity, besides which, their true initial point may be recognized in passing the naked ear, then the stethoscope, successively from the point where the sound is heard, up to the heart, and back again. If the pulsation arises from aneurism of the aorta, it will grow weaker as we approach the heart, and *vice versa.* Aneurism of the descending aorta, may be recognized by a simple, strong pulsation, distinct from the double pulsation of the heart, and from the fact that this latter never extends itself with similar intensity, as far as the back, besides which a rasping or bellows murmur will be heard and abnormal dulness perceived.

Asthma.

§ 277. Shortness of breath, produced by certain diseases of the pulmonary or circulatory organs, sometimes extends to the degree of asthma, a disease which in itself, is a disqualification for the military service. When asthma is thus dependent upon organic lesion, it is ordinarily continuous, although varying in intensity according to circumstances. The examining surgeon can consequently witness its manifestations, and comparing its symptoms with the other signs of visceral alteration, he will find, in their combination, the basis for his opinion. He should above all things, not omit an examination of the lungs, heart, and aorta. There is, however, a species of asthma (nervous asthma), which belongs to no organic lesion, and which only reveals itself, ordinarily, by nocturnal paroxysms of variable frequency. Among soldiers the reality of this disease, which cannot be feigned, may be ascertained in the hospital; but it should never be admitted in the case of recruits, except upon proof obtained for that purpose.

SECTION XXXIV.

DISEASES OF THE SPINE.

Deformities.

§ 278. Deformities of the spine originate either in an organic alteration of the vertebræ themselves, or in a defective equilibrium between the different motor forces, which act upon the column which they compose.

Curvatures of the Spine.

§ 279. These deformities may be either congenital, acquired, or symptomatic of Potts' disease. The spinal column, under the influence of the forces which move it, may be curved forward, backward, or laterally. Such deformities involve absolute incapacity for the duties of a soldier, either because they may compress the spinal cord, and give rise consecutively, to alterations in functions over which this organ presides; or they may interrupt the action of the thoracic viscera, and predispose them to serious lesions; or finally, because they deprive the soldier of the freedom and precision of those movements which are necessary, and because they also occasion great hindrance to equipments. But the different curvatures spoken of may be feigned or artificially produced. Men occasionally present themselves with excessive curvature of the spine, the chest hollowed in, and pretending that they are unable to straighten themselves. This cheat may be exposed, either by placing the man on the floor, face downwards, tightly compressing his loins with a belt, and then stretching his arms out over his head; or else, placing him upon his back, and removing all points of support for his extremities.

Lateral curvatures are more easily feigned. They may be imitated through muscular action alone, by assisting this with mechanical agents, tending either to curve directly the vertebral axis, or to displace the relations of the pelvis, and consequently those of the flexible column which it supports, together with the centre of gravity. Such may be the success, that the simulator, contrary to his intention, remains permanently humpbacked, and this, too, without any advantage, for it is not impossible to distinguish feigned or artificially-produced curvatures from spontaneous ones. The latter, as a first characteristic, have a tendency to attack a variety of points, and to assume a variety of forms, and being as diversified as the particular cases themselves, may occupy any region of the spine. Again, no real deformity of any extent is ever seen having but one curvature; there are always two or three, and sometimes four alternately, when they are produced in order to maintain, by counterbalancing, the axis of the trunk in the line of gravity. Each curvature is always accompanied by a twisting movement of the vertebræ, proportional to its arc and chord. This torsion impresses upon the muscular prominences, on either side of the median line, at the projections of the ribs and shoulders, a noticeable want of symmetry, according to the number, the seat, and the degree of the curvatures. At each curvature, there is a corresponding elevation of the muscles of the ribs and of the shoulder-blade of the convex side, while the concavity is marked by a depression of all its included parts. There are no furrows formed by the wrinkling of the skin, unless the deformity is very extensive, and then they are ordinarily shallow, on account of the retraction of the skin, which in the end always effaces them. These furrows occur in the majority of instances, just below the axilla, and then the chief curvature has its convexity on the opposite side, and in the dorsal region. If, as an extraordinary thing, they are located between the floating ribs and the crest of the ilium, there will be a dorso-lumbar curvature, with extensive uplifting of the ribs and muscles, corresponding to the convexity. There may finally exist a well-marked furrow on a level with a lumbar curvature, without extensive torsion of the vertebræ included in that region, while another furrow corresponds on the opposite side to the dorsal curvature. In such an exceptional case, the dorsal curvature is extensive, descends to the last vertebræ of this region, and is accompanied by a high degree of torsion which raises the last ribs, and produces a depression, with wrinkling of the skin, above the crest of the ilium. Hence, in those rare cases where the real deformity is accompanied by wrinkles of the skin, there is necessarily extensive curvature, and torsion of one or the other side, with consecutive bulging of the muscles and ribs, and lateral, dorsal, or lumbar deformity. Finally, if the hips are no longer on a level, one never differs from the other by more than a few lines, unless there be proportional inequality in the length of the lower limbs.

When the disease is feigned, whatever may be the

means employed, the same external appearance is always remarked, viz.: a single lateral curvature, describing a regular arc, which invariably includes the dorsal and lumbar regions, with lateral inclination of the column upon the pelvis; and such is the sameness and uniformity with which these effects constantly reproduce themselves, that it is next to impossible not to recognize the fraud. The trunk is more or less inclined to the side opposite the convexity, according as the pelvis is more or less elevated on this side, or depressed upon the other. The degree of curvature, which takes place on a large radius, is not in harmony with the degree of inclination of the trunk, whose superior extremity departs widely from the vertical line, this inclination not being counterbalanced by any counter curvature. Within this curvature, and between the floating ribs and the crest of the ilium, the skin of the hip exhibits two or three parallel folds, the shoulder of the side corresponding to the convexity is much more elevated than the other, but both exhibit the same prominence in the rear, together with the ribs, and the two surfaces of corresponding muscles; in other words, there is no trace of torsion. The hips, according to the means employed, may remain on a level, or that of the concave side be raised from two to three and a half inches, and in such case, the corresponding limb appears proportionally shortened; there is also a semblance of limping, which does not occur in the real deformity. These curvatures can only be maintained by the exclusive power of the will, during standing, sitting, or marching.

They may also, when long maintained by mechanical agents, continue permanent, and constitute a real exciting cause whose effects vary, according to the agencies employed in its production, and which it is here needless to enumerate. It suffices to say that:

1st. When it has not been protracted, the action of these agencies, impresses upon the spine none of those characteristics of multiple or alternative curvature, and of torsion of the vertebræ, which distinguish true deformities.

2d. Even after their application, and their long-continued use, the most ingeniously combined means of provocation, although they may have occasioned alternating curvatures, yet do not produce torsion, and reveal through this fact, and the special, always identical form of the curvature, the means of distinguishing the feigned from the real disease.

The diagnosis being established, if the deformity, whether of spontaneous or provoked origin, has now become permanent, the party must be rejected or discharged.

Potts' Disease.

§ 280. This affection is one of very serious consesequence, in a military point of view. It reveals itself by a prominence and bulging of the spinous process, corresponding to the vertebra which is its seat, and sometimes by the presence of cold abscesses, at varying distances from this point. In its incipient stage patients are themselves often ignorant of the existence of local lesion, and do not complain of these secondary effects. In order to discover the disease, the patient must be made to bend forward, while the hand is passed over the spine, to test its sensibility, and to examine critically any abnormal protuberances or depressions which may be encountered. There can be no doubt as to the decision proper in such cases.

Abscess.

§ 281. Large dorsal abscess, if it does not terminate by resolution, may occasion the most serious consequences, by reason of the suppuration which accompanies it. It should always be a cause for rejection, and often for discharge.

Carbuncle.

§ 282. Of the various tumors which may occur in the back, we shall only mention *anthrax*, or carbuncle, as among those often seen, and which should cause rejection, when extensive; but would only justify a discharge through its possible consequences.

SECTION XXXV.

DISEASES OF THE LUMBAR REGION AND OF THE ABDOMEN.

§ 283. Partly connected with diseases of the back, especially with its deformities, diseases of the loins are yet, on many accounts, entirely distinct from them, in a military point of view.

Spina Bifida.

§ 284. The only deformity deserving of notice, on account of the special character of its seat, is hydrorachitis, or spina bifida, which is congenital, and sometimes continues up to puberty, though very rarely, up to adult age. It constitutes an absolute disqualification for the duties of a soldier.

Lumbago.

§ 285. Lumbar rheumatism, or lumbago, is usually a trifling affection, yet it sometimes masks serious disease, either of the spinal column, of the cord, or of the kidneys. It becomes therefore necessary to explore its seat with the greatest attention, in order to establish a correct diagnosis, and not to confound these pains with ostitis, caries, necrosis, or disease of the kidney.

The surgeon should always remember, that chronic rheumatism is often feigned; whence the greater reason for examining carefully the region in which it is alleged to exist. When the disease is real, whether it be a rheumatism, or a more serious lesion, the lower limbs are frequently wasted, with more or less paralysis of sensation or motion, and traces of the external treatment, to which they have been subjected, by leeches, cups, moxas, cauterizations, &c., may at times be discovered. These cases, when well marked, always require the rejection, and frequently the discharge of a party.

Lumbar Hernias.

§ 286. Lumbar hernias are very rare; still, it is well to understand their possibility, and to be able to diagnosticate them.

Psoas Abscess.

§ 287. Psoitis, or inflammation of the psoas muscle, is a serious disease, rarely terminating in resolution. The two foregoing diseases are always causes for rejection, and frequently for discharge.

Diseases of the Abdomen.

§ 288. The abdomen, in its normal state, should be

uniformly soft and elastic, moderately developed, and exhibit no irregular prominences, either externally, or on palpation, however deeply pressure may be made. Exploration by palpation, is extremely important, whenever the complexion of the skin, or any peculiarity in the external appearance, suggests the existence of visceral lesion. Percussion, with whose details the physician should be familiar, also furnishes important indications. (*Vide* Auscultatory-Percussion Chart.)

Contusions.

§ 289. Contusions of the abdomen may produce effects of variable intensity. Their consequences, in the form of ecchymosis, whether circumscribed or diffused, occasionally give rise to extensive abscesses, which spread between the muscular or superficial fascia, and are of very serious character. Whenever such a case presents itself, particular attention must be given to the extent of the ecchymosis, the depth of the contusion, the seat, nature, and intensity of the pain experienced, and whether constantly, or only on pressure. There can be no doubt as to the proper decision, whenever the diagnosis shows that the contusion has involved the internal viscera, stomach, bowels, liver, spleen, &c.

Traumatic Peritonitis.

§ 290. Local traumatic peritonitis, being liable to be followed by serious disorders, even involving life, such as adhesions, internal strangulations, &c., &c., is a cause for rejection, wherever it may be situated.

Wounds.

§ 291. Non-penetrating wounds of the abdomen are

of trifling importance, unless they have been followed by loss of substance, weakening its walls, and predisposing to hernias or adherent cicatrices. These last always constitute a cause for rejection, and often for discharge. The same decision applies to scars following surgical operations. *Penetrating* wounds acquire their importance from the visceral lesions they occasion, and which are recognized by variable signs, according to the nature and functions of the wounded organs.

Hernia.

§ 292. The umbilicus, the median line, the groin, and the femoral region, are, among men, the most common localities for hernia. Other forms of this disease, though extremely rare, are also known, such, for example, as ischiatic, obturator, diaphragmatic, or lumbar hernias.

Inguinal hernia is much the most common of all. Whether easily reducible or not, recent or of long standing, simple or complicated, every form of abdominal hernia must be considered a cause for rejection, on account of the numerous inconveniences which constantly attend it, and the dangerous complications to which it may give rise ; such, for example, as adhesions, dropsy of the sac, obstruction, inflammation, strangulation, and gangrene—all which are especially liable to occur during the period of life occupied by military ser vice, and to be produced by its various contingencies.

Rejection should even be made of those, who, al though not suffering from complete hernia, yet present a well-marked tendency to it, characterized by the following conditions, viz., dilatation of the inguinal ring; relaxation and weakness of the inguinal canal, together with that of the corresponding portion of the anterior abdominal wall.

This predisposition to hernia, can, at times, only be discovered by a most critical examination; yet the subject is of so much importance as to merit all the attention of the surgeon. When the foregoing characteristics are plainly perceived, they leave no room for doubt. Among soldiers, predisposition alone does not justify a discharge; the existence of the disease must be confirmed, whatever may be its degree, from that of a commencing bubonocele, to complete eventration.

Hernia cannot be feigned. It is well to be reminded, however, that deceivers have sometimes attempted to practise imposition in this particular, by wearing a truss (old or much worn), although no appearance of hernia existed.

Hernia may be concealed; whence it becomes necessary not simply to examine the course of the median line, the inguinal, and crural regions, and to apply the hand over their corresponding openings, while the party is made to cough; but also, in pushing up the scrotum, to carry the finger into the inguinal ring, in order to ascertain the fact of its dilatation, and whether some portion of viscera, descending into the canal, does not present itself at the orifice. It is well, also, to make the party lift a weight at arm's length.

Fistulas and Artificial Anus.

§ 293. Abdominal fistulas are absolute causes for rejection or discharge, whenever they manifestly communicate with the cavity of the peritoneum, or one of the viscera. Hence, simple, serous, or puriform fistulas, consequent upon the presence of foreign bodies, or an accidental perforation, produce this double consequence, less from the fact of the fistula itself, than from its origin, and the chronic character of the disease upon which it depends. The same rule will apply, for a much stronger reason, to compound fistulas, having their seat in some particular region of the abdomen, and originating either in the stomach or intestinal canal, and permitting the escape of alimentary, chylous, or fæcal substances; these last form, when narrow, stercoral fistulas, and constitute, when large, the disgusting infirmity known as *artificial anus*, an opening sometimes of accidental and traumatic nature, or resulting from gangrene of a strangulated hernia—sometimes artificially produced, in order to remedy an intestinal obliteration, either congenital or acquired.

The same rule will apply to hepatic, or biliary fistulas, which are very rare; as also to urinary fistulas of the kidney or bladder.

Tumors.

§ 294. Palpation and percussion serve to discover deep-seated tumors, enlargement of the liver and spleen, which are chronic lesions, with or without general constitutional symptoms indicating their severity, but whose presence leaves no doubt as to the disqualification of their subjects. Nevertheless, when such tumors exhibit themselves in soldiers, no discharge should be granted, until treatment has proved unavailing.

Simple stercoral tumors, the nature of which it is very important to recognize, are not, properly speaking, a disease.

Inguinal Tumors.—Deep-seated Abscess.

§ 295. Deep-seated abscess of the iliac fossa, is always

a cause for rejection. Inguinal abscesses are often symptomatic of caries; they are at times stercoral or urinary. All these affections, which necessitate both rejection and discharge, might, through carelessness, be mistaken for hernia.

Adenitis.

§ 296. Inguinal adenitis is frequent, and often of syphilitic origin. When associated with enlarged cervical glands, it indicates scrofula, or syphilis, and may require the rejection of a party, through the diseased bodily condition which it reveals.

Infra-inguinal adenitis is symptomatic of superficial mechanical lesions of the leg, or foot, and may be looked upon as a trifling disease.

Syphilitic Adenitis (venereal bubo) may become a cause for rejection or discharge, according to the extent and severity of the constitutional symptoms which it has occasioned.

By means of an insufflation of air into the cellular tissue, an inguinal tumor might be produced, but only so as to deceive a superficial observer.

Chronic Inflammations.

§ 297. Chronic inflammations of the stomach, bowels, or peritoneum, invariably exhibit a series of symptoms, which it is useless to rehearse in this connection. These diseases, although often curable, always constitute a cause for rejection. They justify a discharge only when treatment has proved unavailing.

Distension.

§ 298. Many of the foregoing diseases occasion a distension of the abdomen, or tympanitis, which has sometimes been imitated by individuals, possessed of the rare faculty of swallowing air in sufficient quantity to produce enormous distension of the abdomen. Palpation and percussion will generally suffice to determine its cause.

Vomiting at Will.

§ 299. Other persons naturally possess, or have acquired, the faculty of vomiting at will, and endeavor, by this means, to appear as if suffering under chronic lesion of the stomach.

Hæmatemesis.

§ 300. Others, again, complain of habitual vomiting of blood, and in order to make good their assertion, feign this hæmorrhage by ejecting, in the presence of the surgeon, a quantity of blood, secretly swallowed beforehand. In all these cases which, if real, would necessarily be complicated with marked constitutional disturbance, the general bodily condition of the parties, and absence of emaciation—two unequivocal signs of health—would strongly testify against their allegations.

Hypertrophy of the Liver and Spleen.

§ 301. Chronic enlargement of the liver, cancer, abscess, and hydatids which often have their seat there, when proved to exist, are causes for rejection or discharge.

Abscess of the Spleen.

§ 302. The same rule will apply to abscesses of the spleen, which are rare, and to its abnormal enlargement (ague-cake), which accompanies, nearly always, malarious cachexy. Nevertheless, the last named does not justify a discharge, until curative treatment has proved unavailing.

In malarious districts, slight hypertrophy of the abdominal viscera cannot be considered a disqualifying circumstance, since removal from the sources of endemic influence, is the most successful method of overcoming it, as happens with those removed from *goitrous localities*. Changes of climate, modifications of diet, and removal of the exciting cause, generally restore the organ to its natural state. In particular instances great attention should be paid to the general bodily condition of the party; his local disease is only a subordinate consideration.

Biliary Calculi.

§ 303. Calculous tumors of the gall-bladder are absolute causes for rejection or discharge.

Icterus (Jaundice).

§ 304. Jaundice is of varying importance, according as it is idiopathic, or symptomatic of disease of the liver. In the former case, it is a trifling and temporary disease; in the latter case, the decision must be based upon the original disease, as presumed or recognized. Jaundice may be clumsily feigned, but the sclerotic could not be colored, and this circumstance alone would suffice to expose the cheat.

Tænia (Tape-worm).

§ 305. *Tænia*, and other intestinal worms, are not a cause either for rejection or discharge.

SECTION XXXVI.

DISEASES OF THE PELVIS.

Congenital Deformities.

§ 306. Congenital deformities of the pelvis are rare among men; nevertheless it may be of inordinate size or extreme narrowness. These organic conditions justify the rejection of a party, whenever they are sufficiently marked to exercise any influence upon the internal organs or the lower limbs.

Relaxation of the Symphyses.

§ 307. Among mechanical lesions, need only be cited relaxations of the symphyses, which may follow certain forms of external violence, and constitute an absolute disqualification for the duties of a soldier.

Sprain or Luxation of the Os-Coccygis.

§ 308. Sprain or luxation of the coccyx being easily reducible, and leaving no consequences, would only justify rejection in very exceptional cases.

Wounds.

§ 309. Accidental or artificial wounds of the perineum, if they remain fistulous or unhealed, constitute, in such case alone, a cause for rejection; but not for discharge, unless they are of long standing, or complicated with other lesions.

Lacerations.

§ 310. Lacerations of the perineum are the result, in

men, of external violence, and are ordinarily so slight and superficial, as to leave no results disqualifying a party for military service. The presence of any evidence of past extensive contusions should occasion an examination for stricture.

Fistulas.

§ 311. Fistulas, resulting from mechanical lesions, surgical operations, or open tumors in this region, are either purulent, stercoral, or urinary; each one distinguishing itself by special signs, which can leave no doubt as to the proper decision to be given.

Tumors.

§ 312. The tumors most common to this region are the hæmatic, resulting from contusions or collections of blood, pus, or fæces; abscesses depending upon caries of the ischium, calculous tumors (rare), and perineal hernia, properly so called (not less rare), formed between the rectum and the bladder, and requiring careful exploration to discover it. These tumors, which cannot be feigned, and are of difficult treatment, always constitute a cause for rejection; their degree of development will indicate the necessity for a discharge.

SECTION XXXVII.

DISEASES OF THE ANUS AND RECTUM.

§ 313. The lower part of the rectum and the anus are, of all portions of the bowels, those which present the greatest number of diseases deserving the attention of examining surgeons. A critical examination of this orifice, of the folds of the sphincter, and of the discharges liable to flow from these parts, should be made. Many of the diseases having their seat there can be feigned, which affords an additional reason for paying the greatest attention to their diagnosis.

Traumatic Lesions.

§ 314. Contused wounds, lacerations, and perforations of the anus and rectum, are at times followed by deep cicatrices, or, on the contrary, by incomplete cicatrization, which may occasion either retention or incontinence of fæces. Rejection of the party should be made, only when well-marked signs of one or the other of these conditions are established.

Foreign Bodies.

§ 315. Foreign bodies originally swallowed, and lodging in the rectum, or introduced there, accidentally or wilfully, can ordinarily be extracted. They serve at times to counterfeit diseased conditions which it is always necessary to recognize.

Worms.

§ 316. As to those verminous affections which have their seat near the anal orifice, they afford neither cause for rejection nor discharge.

Syphilis.

§ 317. Syphilitic diseases of the rectum and anus, such as purulent discharge, ulcerations, fissures, mucous pustules, condylomata, and warty growths, are curable in common with the parent disease, and therefore not incompatible with the duties of a soldier.

Various Affections, Fistulas, &c.

§ 318. The same rule will apply to simple inflammation of the anus, to simple neuralgia, and furunculous or idiopathic abscesses of the margin of the anus. But deep-seated abscesses, or those symptomatic of caries of the sacrum or ischium, simple fistula ani, if complete, are causes for rejection and sometimes for discharge.

Spasmodic contraction and fissures of the anus, spasmodic contraction of the sphincter ani, when existing in a simple state, cannot be recognized by the examining surgeon, because no positive sign, appreciable to the senses, accompanies it. Spasmodic stricture, dependent upon fissure, or irritable ulcer, will most ordinarily be distinguished with ease by the recognition of the fissure itself, whose lower extremity can be generally detected by separating the folds of the anus. These affections, which are not very common among young men, should be considered in the light of inconveniences rather than diseases. They always yield to a simple surgical operation which the patient can long avoid, if he prefers to suffer during, and for some time after, defecation. Consequently, simple spasm of the anus never is a cause either for rejection or discharge; fissure could only justify rejection, if very deep, multiple, of malignant aspect, and particularly if connected with some existing lesion of the lungs. It should never authorize a discharge until, by its complications, it has successfully resisted all surgical treatment.

Stricture of the Rectum, Cancer, &c.

§ 319. The anus and the rectum are, to a distance within reach of the finger, sometimes narrowed by hard, scirrhus, annular swellings, or by tumors, of various nature, arising from the walls of the bowel, or acting upon these by compression from without. When these diseases exist about the anus, or have extended to its orifice, they are easily recognized by sight and touch; at other times, touch, combined with the speculum, can alone establish the existence of the disease. In such case, if the interior of the bowel is explored, there will be felt at more or less distance from, sometimes at the anus itself, a resistant ring, of fibrous character, which it is impossible or very difficult to pass. Manipulation is at times painful, at other times nearly imperceptible. The diseased part is occasionally smooth, hard as it were, callous, and covered with granulations, which the least touch causes to bleed. The altered portion appears movable and surrounded by healthy, and detached cellular tissue. These diseases are always of serious character, and afford, when well marked, causes for both rejection and discharge.

Hæmorrhoids.

§ 320. The anus may be the seat of hæmorrhoids, which in the form of internal or external tumors, ulcerated or not, are a cause for rejection; while they do not necessarily justify a discharge. In the latter case, collateral circumstances should guide the judgment, as well as the principal fact. It will be necessary therefore, to investigate the amount of inconvenience which it causes in defecation; and, under other circumstances, the influence of the loss of blood upon the general economy, the amount of prolapsus, the difficulty experienced in reducing the tumor, together with its liability to come down, upon exertion. These considerations will determine the expediency of retaining or discharging a soldier. As to periodical loss of blood, without either internal or external tumor, it affords no ground for rejection, until shown to exist by indubitable proofs, such as anæmia, &c. It is unnecessary to mention the gross practices by which hæmorrhoids are feigned, as they never can deceive an examining surgeon.

Procidentia of the Mucous Membrane, and Prolapsus of the Rectum.

§ 321. Old ulcerated piles, or other causes, such as extensive relaxation, or loss of substance, or paralysis of the sphincters and levator ani, may occasion procidentia of the mucous membrane of the rectum through the anus. The importance of this disease varies according as the tumor is reducible after defecation, by the patient himself, or is large, difficult to return, and to maintain within the anus; liable to reappear on slight effort being made, or continues permanently external, which then constitutes prolapsus of the rectum. Simple procidentia, which does not effect the general health, is not a cause for rejection or discharge. But permanent prolapsus of the rectum always constitutes an absolute disqualification for the duties of a soldier.

Incontinence of Fæces.

§ 322. Whether or not, accompanied by prolapsus, paralysis of the rectum always occasions incontinence of fæces, and besides, is generally complicated with other serious disorders, producing similar disqualifications in its subjects.

SECTION XXXVIII.

DISEASES OF THE URINARY PASSAGES AND ORGANS.

Incontinence of Urine.

§ 323. Diseases of the urinary passages, which should be studied in the light of possible obstacles to the discharge of a soldier's duties, are not less numerous nor less important than those of preceding regions.

Incontinence of urine although rare, is often alleged before examining surgeons. It may be considered feigned, whenever it cannot be explained by an abnormal and excessive dilatation of the urethra, by the presence of vesical calculus, by external traces of a serious wound, or operation, or when it is unaccompanied by a feeble and prostrated condition of the system, forming of itself, a disqualification for the duties of a soldier. The sexual organs and the surrounding parts present a peculiar aspect in the really incontinent, and which is not met with in malingerers. It is moreover easy to detect this simulation when it applies to *permanent* incontinence. In such cases it is only necessary to cause the patient to pass water, and to notice how it escapes from the meatus; if the incontinence is real, the urine passes drop by drop, precisely as secreted, and without any effort on the part of the subject, or muscular contraction; in the opposite case, the urine passes with a sensible jet, and by means of efforts which it is easy to notice. *Nocturnal* incontinence presents more difficulties, because alleged to occur only during sleep. But an acquaintance with the various causes of real incontinence, enables one, in most instances, to discover the signs of the affection when feigned. These causes, frequently of mechanical origin, depend upon an accidental lesion or a local affection of the bladder, or the urethra; or else are symptomatic of alterations of vital properties, following, for example, certain acute diseases with nervous prostration; or arise simply from weakness and relaxation of the neck of the bladder. Deception can nearly always be discovered by placing the subject at bedtime under the influence of opium, having first disposed him to drink copiously through the day, by strongly salting his food. On visiting him during the night, his bed will not always be found wet, and on emptying the bladder with a sound, more or less urine will be drawn off.

Finally, incontinence, when purely symptomatic of well-marked local disease, is always a cause for rejection, and often for discharge. But the same is not the case with permanent or nocturnal incontinence, because this disease, which is very rare, as before said, resulting, in most cases, from indolence and defective training, is, in general, easily curable by means of vigilant supervision, even if it does not terminate spontaneously.

Retention of Urine.

§ 324. Retention of urine, of which dysuria is only a minor degree, notwithstanding its frequency and serious character, rarely comes before examining surgeons. Yet, at times, it is seen when in an incipient stage, or when disposed to yield to regular catheterism. It may be feigned, or artificially produced; but with difficulty, since the least pressure on the hypogastric region would tend to overpower the resistance or contraction of the neck of the bladder, and to empty it instantly.

The protuberance formed by the distended bladder might be mistaken for another disease, as for example, an encysted tumor, or even ascites. Catheterism will at once determine the diagnosis. But if the obstacle to passing water arises from an organic cause, and particularly from stricture of the urethra—a rather rare thing among young men—the retention, whether actually existing, or only possible, is a cause for rejection. This disease is too often curable to justify a discharge, unless in very exceptional cases.

Diabetes.

§ 325. Well-marked diabetes is an absolute cause for rejection or discharge. But this complex disease, of rather rare occurrence in young men, may present at the outset doubtful signs, and such as are difficult to recognize.*

* The following tests are easily applied to diabetic urine, and should be accordingly resorted to:

Moore's test.—Boil equal quantities of the suspected urine and liquor potassæ, in a test-tube, when, if diabetes exist, the solution assumes a claret color, of more or less depth, according to the quantity of sugar present.

Trommer's test.—In a large test-tube, mix, with some of the suspected urine, just enough of a solution of sulphate of copper to give it a faint blue tint. Then add liquor potassæ in considerable excess. If sugar be present, a precipitate of hydrated oxide of copper first falls, which is redissolved in the excess of alkali, forming a dark blue solution. If this be gently heated to ebullition, a dense deposit of red suboxide of copper takes place.

Hæmaturia.

§ 326. Hæmaturia, or bloody urine, is rather a serious disease whenever it originates in the kidneys or in the bladder, and is not simply of a temporary character. It is of rare occurrence, however, among young men. Besides traumatic causes, hæmaturia may result from the suppression of an habitual hæmorrhage, epistaxis for example, or depend, although more rarely, upon a scorbutic affection, or the hæmorrhagic diathesis. In these cases, rejection or discharge must follow.

Albuminuria.

§ 327. Albuminuria, which can be certainly ascertained by the use of proper means, is an absolute disqualification for the duties of a soldier.*

Urinary Calculi.

§ 328. Urinary calculi, whether originating in the kidney, under the form of *gravel*, or whether formed in the bladder, or lodging themselves in the prostate or the urethra, present ordinarily very characteristic signs, but which nevertheless require an attentive examination. Their presence, when well established, requires the rejection of a party, and even his discharge, if he will not submit to the necessary operations.

Urinary Abscesses.

§ 329. Urinary abscesses and fistulas, whatever may be their seat, always require the rejection of a party, and his discharge, when the complications of the fistula necessitate a long treatment whose results are uncertain.

* Heat, nitric acid, and microscopical examinations of the urinary sediments, will determine the existence of this disease.

Mechanical Lesions of the Kidneys.

§ 330. Diseases of the kidney require practical experience in palpation and percussion, the sources which, together with microscopical examinations of the urinary sediments, furnish the principal signs of their existence. Congenital lesions of the kidney are not amenable to examination.

These organs may, in common with the others, be the seat of various mechanical lesions, such as contusions and concussions, which it is often difficult to discover, and wounds or lacerations, which frequently require the rejection of a party, though more rarely his discharge. Foreign bodies, introduced by external violence, may remain lodged in their substance. Whenever their presence is recognized, they constitute an absolute incapacity for the duties of a soldier.

Nephritis.

§ 331. Inflammation of the kidneys, of which it is important to establish the diagnosis, in order not to mistake it for diseases of less gravity (such as lumbago), may be simple, traumatic, albuminous, calculous, rheumatic, gouty, or purulent (the result of resorption), in character. These all constitute causes for rejection, and often for discharge.

Renal Calculi.

§ 332. Urinary calculi, which are suspected, for the most part, only from the violent pains attending them, particularly in their passage through the ureters, but of which no certainty exists until their escape from the urethra, are always a cause for rejection or discharge.*

* The fact of having once passed a urinary calculus does not afford presumptive evidence that another is likely to follow, or the diathesis to continue, upon which its existence depends.

Abscesses.—Fistulas.

§ 333. Renal abscesses and fistulas, tumors, cysts, and cancer, are causes for rejection, but not necessarily for discharge.

Diseases of the Bladder.

§ 334. The importance of the bladder is such, that all diseases capable of affecting it are of a serious character, and deserve particular attention; nor are they the less worthy of study on account of their extreme frequency.

An examination of this organ by direct palpation will reveal its condition of fulness or emptiness; catheterism alone can give correct ideas of some of the lesions of which it is the seat; while examination of its excretions is indispensable as a means of diagnosis.

Absence of the Bladder.—Extrophia (extroversion).

§ 335. Complete absence of the bladder is very rare; yet it has been observed.

Extrophia, or extroversion, of this organ, exhibits itself in the form of a loss of substance of the inferior portion of the walls of the abdomen, and by the presence of a red, moist surface, on which the ureters are sometimes seen, allowing the urine to escape directly.

Atrophy of the bladder has occasionally been mistaken for its absence.

The foregoing diseases are all manifest disqualifications for the military service.

Hypertrophy.

§ 336. The bladder may also be hypertrophied, and occupy a large space in the abdomen. It may also open into various abnormal localities through imperforations of the ureters, as for example, through the umbilicus with persistence of the urachus, or through the rectum. These cases are extremely rare; still, it is well to be apprised of their possibility. It is almost needless to add, that they constitute a cause for rejection.

Traumatic Lesions.

§ 337. The bladder may be the seat of contusions, of compressions, if full, of rupture, and of wounds of various nature, particularly gunshot. These lesions are so immediately serious in their nature as rarely to come before examining surgeons. If any should present themselves, they would constitute a cause for rejection, but not of discharge, until surgical treatment had proved unavailing.

Foreign bodies sometimes find their way into the bladder, either through wounds or catheterism (fragments of a sound). These form constant causes for rejection, but not of discharge, until all attempts at extraction have proved abortive, or serious disorders have been produced by such bodies.

Vesical Calculi.

§ 338. Vesical calculi reveal their presence by pain, a sense of weight at the lower part of the bladder, turbid urine, sometimes purulent, sometimes sanguinolent, intermission in the flow of the urine, and pain at the extremity of the penis; but the only true pathognomonic sign is furnished by the sound.

Paralysis.

§ 339. Paralysis of the bladder, of which atony constitutes the first stage, arises nearly always from lesion of some other organ, particularly of the spinal cord.

This disease, of easy recognition, by its own characteristics, and those of its parent source, derives all its importance from the diseased condition of the latter.

Cystitis.

§ 340. Inflammation of the bladder, whether acute or chronic, is always a sufficiently serious disease to require the rejection of a party. Nevertheless, it must be borne in mind that this disease may be artificially produced by partaking of certain substances well known to physicians. It is, therefore, important to assure one's self that the inflammation is not due to this cause, for in such case it is trifling, and occasions no disqualification.

Hydatids.

§ 341. Hydatids, although rare, are at times met with in the bladder. Their presence, when duly established, constitutes a disqualification for the duties of a soldier.

Vesical Fistulas.

§ 342. Gangrene, wounds, operations for puncture, or lithotomy, sometimes leave behind them urinary fistulas, which are always a cause for rejection.

Hernia.

§ 343. Hernia of the bladder may occur in various directions, constituting either abdominal, inguinal, or perineal cystocele. These are all causes for rejection or discharge. The same rule will apply to a varicose state of the neck of the bladder, to polypi, fungous growths, etc., which are at times observed, though very rarely in young men.

Diseases of the Urethra.

§ 344. It is more particularly to diseases of the urethra, that catheterism applies as a means of diagnosis. Direct examination by the hand must not be neglected, as it enables us to discover foreign bodies lodged in the corpus cavernosum, together with any protuberances formed by structural alterations.

Simple inspection suffices to detect diseases situated in the vicinity of the meatus; while a catheter or sound is necessary to explore the deeper portions of this canal.

Anomalies.

§ 345. The urethra may be entirely wanting, imperforate, or turned from its normal direction. The two first anomalies would require the rejection or discharge of a party, while a simple deviation might not.

Hypospadias.

§ 346. The urine may be voided in an abnormal way, as, for example, in hypospadias, epispadias, and fistulas. In hypospadias, the opening occurs either at the fossa navicularis, near to, or corresponding with, the frænum of the prepuce, or between this point and the scrotum, or in the scrotum itself.

In epispadias, the orifice is near the root, and on the dorsum of the penis, which organ is slightly developed, and most often cleft throughout its entire length.

Hypospadias is not a disqualification for military service, whenever the opening is situated at the extremity of the penis, beneath the gland, and the urine can be ejected to some distance; when, in fact, the opening is large enough to permit the escape of a stream of urine of normal size, which may be ascertained by a bougie, or causing the subject to pass water before the surgeon. In all other cases, there is a total disqualification for the military service. A person, laboring under such infirmities, cannot avoid soiling his garments during every passage of water, and these soon become offensive, to an intolerable degree, to all about him; while the humidity itself is a source of constant danger to his health. The same rule necessarily applies to urinary fistulas, with this difference, that when they occur in soldiers, an operation should first be resorted to, wherever the case justifies it, before granting a discharge.

Foreign Bodies.

§ 347. Foreign bodies are occasionally introduced into the urethra either accidentally or through design; these bodies, not admitting of being extracted without a surgical operation, afford a cause for rejection. Calculi, lodging themselves there, would produce a similar disqualification, not only as being foreign bodies, but because they would create fears of the presence of other calculi in the kidneys or bladder. On the other hand, they would afford a cause for discharge, only in exceptional cases.

Stricture.

§ 348. Strictures of the urethra, recognizable by the bougie, or by causing the subject to pass water in one's presence (the stream of urine is often in such cases forked or twisted) is a disease of difficult cure, and productive of consequences incompatible with the discharge of a soldier's duties. Nevertheless, whenever it occurs in a soldier, no discharge should be granted until all curative means have failed.

8*

Urethritis.

§ 349. Inflammation of the urethra, whether acute or chronic, never is a cause for rejection or discharge.

Diseases of the Prostate.

§ 350. Diseases of the prostate are very rare among young men. This gland may be the seat of hypertrophy, either congenital or acquired; of various mechanical lesions, or of calculous disease. The decision to be arrived at in each case must be determined by the nature of the lesions, which may be either trifling and without importance, or seriously endanger the functions of the organ. Young men often believe themselves the subjects of serious diseases of the prostate, when, in fact, none exist. In such cases, they should always be subjected to a manual examination by the rectum.

SECTION XXXIX.

DISEASES OF THE GENITAL ORGANS.

§ 351. The frequency and variety of the diseases of the genital organs in man, require the closest attention, and a certain amount of practical experience, when viewed in the light of causes for rejection or discharge. Some of these diseases exhibit forms or degrees at times incompatible with the discharge of a soldier's duties.

Traumatic Lesions.

§ 352. Accidental mutilations of the genital organs,

occasioning complete or almost entire loss of these parts, whether arising from criminal acts, particularly with cutting instruments, or from gunshot wounds, require both the rejection and the discharge of a party. In fact, the loss of these parts becomes at once a cause of physical infirmity (with obstacle to passing water or complication of fistulas) and a cause of moral infirmity, through the depressive influences which belong to this infirmity. But the same is not the case in partial lesions, or such as are capable of being cured.

DISEASES OF THE PENIS.

Phymosis and Paraphymosis.

§ 353. Phymosis and paraphymosis, existing without complication, are not a cause either for rejection or discharge, since they can always be readily cured. The simple operation for phymosis has sometimes sufficed to remove symptoms which were attributed to the presence of vesical calculus.

Atrophy.

§ 354. Atrophy of the penis, however marked, is not a cause for rejection, unless accompanied by simultaneous atrophy of the testicles. But extensive hypertrophy of this organ, to the degree of constituting elephantiasis, would be a disqualification in itself, as well on account of its tendency to invade the scrotum, as of interfering with marching.

Loss of the Penis.

§ 355. Total, or almost entire, loss of the penis, whether resulting from voluntary mutilation, accidental wounding, or surgical amputation, requires the rejection or discharge of a party. The same rule obtains in cases of crushing of the penis, followed by deformity, rupture of the corpora cavernosa, laceration, fistula, and stricture of the urethra.

Various Affections.

§ 356. As to ulcers, chancres, and syphilitic warts, they do not, in the majority of cases, require any mention here; but it will be different if the penis has been partly destroyed by a phagedenic ulceration, the cure of which would not restore the organ to its natural shape.

DISEASES OF THE SCROTUM.

Wounds.—Lacerations.

§ 357. Wounds or lacerations sufficiently extensive to expose the testicles, may afford causes for rejection. It is well to bear in mind, however, that cicatrization occurs nearly always without adhesions.

Contusions.—Hæmatocele.

§ 358. Violent contusions, or contused wounds, often give rise to hæmatocele by infiltration or extravasation. In the former case (infiltration), the blood is ordinarily absorbed with facility, and rejection is not called for any more than by other forms of ecchymosis, provided there are no complications. This state counterfeits gangrene in a gross way, but the least attention will expose the fallacy. In the latter case (extravasation into the tunica vaginalis), the manifestations bear a strong resemblance to those of hydrocele, and demand a like decision.

Cutaneous Affections.

§ 359. The scrotum may be the seat of various cutaneous affections which spread to the neighboring parts, the internal and superior surface of the thighs, the perineum, and the margin of the anus. These diseases, which are often of difficult cure, and ordinarily provoke an intolerable itching, are aggravated by the friction occasioned by marching, and by the contact of woollen clothing. They constitute a cause for rejection and discharge, under all the conditions mentioned in the chapter devoted to the consideration of these diseases. Care should be taken, however, not to confound them with simple chafing, and other trifling diseases, which do not deserve special mention in this connection.

Swellings and Abscesses.

§ 360. Swellings and abscesses never are a cause for rejection, unless the latter are symptomatic of, or associated with, scrofula.

Urinary Abscesses.

§ 361. Urinary abscesses of the scrotum, are of sufficient importance to constitute a disqualification for the military service.

Emphysema.

§ 362. Air never accumulates in the scrotum. Whenever, therefore, parties present themselves with this region tumefied, light, when compared with its volume—distended, elastic, and resonant under percussion, there is certainly fraud, and the emphysema has been artificially produced.

Œdema.

§ 363. Œdema of the scrotum acquires its importance from the general bodily condition of its subject, and the cause which has originated it. It is never uncomplicated, and this circumstance enables us always to discover the deception, whenever any person has caused water to be injected, through a small opening, into the cellular tissue of the scrotum.

Varicocele.

§ 364. Varicocele, which is a tumor formed by the distension of the spermatic veins, occurring between the external orifice of the inguinal canal and the epididymis, is not a cause for rejection, unless it occasions, by its size, a marked impediment to marching, or the performance of other movements. Nor should a discharge be granted therefor, until curative treatment has proved unavailing. Even then a soldier, if unable to march, may be made useful in some less active capacity.*

* The differential diagnosis of varicocele, and inguinal hernia, is easily established by noticing the following distinctions in their symptoms. In *Hernia*, the tumor is uniformly round, soft, and compressible, and often emits a gurgling sound on pressure; when reduced, it returns on removal of the support and resumption of the upright position, or coughing. In *Varicocele*, the tumor is pyramidal in form, its base resting upon the testis, and its apex ascending into the external ring; it feels like a knot of earthworms (cirsocele), and when reduced, and the patient resumes the upright position, it returns, despite pressure upon the abdominal ring, owing to the circulation continuing in the spermatic veins. This was the test proposed by Sir Astley Cooper. In cases of hernia, the extremity of the finger should be pushed as far as possible into the external abdominal ring, by thrusting the skin of the scrotum before it. Under which circumstances the contact, or impulse of the descending hernia can almost invariably be recognized, when it exists, if the suspected party be made to cough, when in the upright position.

Hydrocele.

§ 365. Hydrocele of the spermatic cord, and that of the tunica vaginalis, are causes for rejection; but not for discharge, inasmuch as its radical cure can be obtained by surgical treatment. It is impossible, in whatever way attempted, to feign, with any degree of probable success, either of these diseases.

Encysted Tumors.—Fistulas.—Calculi.

§ 366. Encysted tumors, of any notable size, by reason of their tendency to increase; fistulas communicating with the tunica vaginalis, or the testicle; calculous concretions of the scrotum, which are rare, are causes for rejection, but not generally for discharge.

Elephantiasis.

§ 367. Hypertrophy of the scrotum and of the subjacent cellular tissue, known as elephantiasis, is extremely rare. But whenever present, would always constitute a cause for rejection.

DISEASES OF THE TESTICLES.

§ 368. The influence exercised by the functional activity of the testicles upon the constitution, the physical and moral courage of individuals, requires that the integrity of these organs should be unimpaired. Hence their loss, atrophy, or the degeneration of either of them, constitutes an absolute incapacity for the military service.

Anorchidia.—Ectopia.

§ 369. Absence of the testicles, or anorchidia, is only apparent; it is often only ectopia, or malposition. Sometimes the testicles have not descended; sometimes, though rarely, they are in the perineum, but more frequently they are lodged in the inguinal canal. Ectopia may be slight, and the testicles capable of being pushed down and maintained there; in which case no cause for rejection would exist. But if they were strongly compressed in the ring, it would be well to reject the party, by reason of the pain they occasion, their tendency to become atrophied, or the hernias to which they often give rise. It is safe to believe in the retention of the testicles in the abdomen, and consequently in the capacity of a party, whenever he exhibits in general, all the other signs of virility, and no credible testimony, nor external signs afford any presumption that these organs have been removed by a surgical operation, or destroyed by wounds.

Atrophy and Loss.

§ 370. Atrophy of the testicles is more often acquired than congenital. It frequently results from premature excesses or mechanical injuries. This condition would not afford any cause for rejection, unless existing to a great degree. Atrophy of one of these organs, the other being healthy and well developed, is not a disqualification for military service; but where the remaining one is attacked, and in an incipient state of atrophy, the party should be rejected.

Orchitis.

§ 371. Inflammations of the testicle may require the rejection of a party, whenever they are the result of considerable violence; and if the disease has become chronic it may also require that a party be discharged. The same rule will apply to syphilitic orchitis, which may be complicated with various consequences, and evince a tendency to degeneration. Gonorrheal epidydimitis, which must not be confounded with the preceding, is not a serious disease, and not likely to lead to any consequences, rendering a party unfit for the duties of a soldier.

Fistulas.

§ 372. The like rule will apply to non-adherent fistulas of the testicles.

Enchondroma.

§ 373. Enchondroma, or cartilaginous degeneration of the testicle, and the other forms of degeneration, of which these organs are frequently the seat, are manifest causes for rejection, and most frequently for discharge.

Diseases of the Spermatic Cord.

§ 374. Chronic inflammation of the spermatic cord, independent of, or complicated with, disease of the testicle, and occasioning either infiltration, or more serious disorders, is a cause for rejection, and sometimes, even for a discharge. The same rule will apply to hydrocele and degeneration, arising from those of the testicle.

Spermatorrhœa.

§ 375. Spermatorrhœa, even if its existence, in an aggravated form, could be demonstrated, should not be a cause for rejection, unless the general health were manifestly broken down, and it were accompanied by evidences of organic disease.

SECTION XL.

DISEASES OF THE LIMBS.

§ 376. Soundness of the limbs, in all their parts, is assuredly one of the most important of all prerequisite conditions for the duties of a soldier. Their shape should exhibit no extremes, either of size, or want of development—the cutaneous functions should be performed with regularity—the perspiration be moderate—the sensibility of touch be normally developed. It is also indispensable that the bony structure should furnish a sufficient fulcrum of resistance to the action of the muscles, and the play of the articulations. Some diseases of the limbs might be concealed and overlooked, if the surgeon neglected to examine in detail the play of all the articulations of the arms, hands, and, in particular, the fingers; and if care were not taken to make the recruit walk.

Anomalies.

§ 377. It is indispensable that both the upper and lower limbs should be mutually alike; every anomaly of organization, therefore, in their number, shape, and relations, is an absolute disqualification for the military service.

Inequality of Limbs.

§ 378. Congenital inequality of the limbs, carried to a marked degree, is very rare. It may be limited to the upper or lower limbs, or extend to both. For example, all the parts of one side have been seen longer, and larger, than those of the other. From such an anomaly there results incapacity for the duties of a soldier; on the one hand, because the manual of arms could not be performed with regularity, by limbs of unequal length and strength; and on the other, because there necessarily results lameness in the lower limbs, with curvature of the spine, and all the inconveniences attendant upon it.

Incurvation of Limbs.

§ 379. Incurvation of the arms is not rare—the fore-arm instead of continuing, in its articulation with the humerus, the almost straight line which the whole arm should make, forms a larger angle, opening outwardly. This deformity may render it impossible to perform, with regularity and precision, certain motions in the handling of arms. The same is the case with bow-legs, which are a disqualification, because they prevent junction of the heels, and occasion an impediment and an irregularity in walking, which extends almost to lameness when the deformity is restricted to one leg. This deformity is, in the majority of cases, associated with scrofula.

Atrophy of the Limbs.

§ 380. Whether atrophy be congenital or acquired, whether it involve all the limbs or be confined to one, the relative weakness which it occasions necessarily constitutes an absolute disqualification for the military service.

Contractions.

§ 381. Contraction, or rigidity, and shortening of certain muscles, with diminution or loss of their normal extensibility, occasions, sometimes flexion, and more rarely permanent extension, of a portion of a limb, and always constitutes an absolute disqualification for the military service. Contraction of limbs is often feigned—a fact which may be suspected whenever it is declared to be of long standing, and yet the limb is not emaciated. There are persons who, for a long while, keep the forearm and leg continually bent, and thus succeed in interrupting the nutrition of their limbs. Others habituate themselves to wearing a high heel, in order to compel flexion of the knee while walking; others, as is most commonly the case, keep the thumb and index finger of one hand in a state of absolute repose, by flexion, or compress the hand with a band, in order to diminish the size of the fingers and to crook them, allowing perspiration and dirt to accumulate beneath them for the purpose of rendering the curvature more probable, and sometimes even burn themselves, in the direction of the tendons of the flexor muscles, to make the retraction appear more natural. All these frauds will fail in the presence of a surgeon enlightened by experience, since the phenomena of nature can never be perfectly imitated by art. In each of the foregoing cases suspicion should be awakened not, properly speaking, when the muscles feel hard and tense alone, as has been said; but when their belly presents, along with hardness, that swelling which accompanies every contraction, and when too there may be felt, within their thickness, those slight jerkings which betray the incessant repetition of contractile efforts on the part of the muscular fasciculi, resisting action imparted to the limb in a different direction. In order to expose the cheat, or to cause suspension of its effects, the simulator must be met by artifice: his attention must be strongly distracted, while at the same time an effort is made to surprise him, and to suddenly overpower resistance. At other times belief must be pretended in his assertions, and he must be led to acts in contradiction with them. Fraud may be discovered by making the suspected man stand on one foot, upon a post slightly elevated, and compelling him to balance himself upon the sound leg; fatigue will soon oblige him to extend the limb artificially contracted. Finally, a more direct and potent expedient offers itself, which consists in applying upon the limb a tight, and well-rolled bandage made of new linen, and afterwards wetting it, in order to increase its compressive power. The limbs being no longer able to contract beneath this uniform impediment, soon cease to resist motion. When the party is in hospital, it will suffice to wait until he is asleep in order to straighten the limb and to expose his deception. This last method of verification is applicable to cases of feigned anchylosis. The use of an anæsthetic will, in general, speedily determine the question.

Supernumerary Limbs.

§ 382. This anomaly is of rare occurrence, so far as it relates to a whole limb. It is sometimes observed, however, with regard to the lower extremities.

It is more frequent when partial and limited, for example, to fingers and toes. Thus, certain persons are born with supernumerary fingers or toes; these may be either rudimentary or possess the complete organization of true fingers or toes. Both these deformities constitute a disqualification for the military service.

Mechanical Lesions.

§ 383. The various mechanical lesions which affect the limbs either in their continuity or their contiguity, deserve serious attention, as well on account of the weakness to which they give rise, as of the deformity which they may occasion. The decision to be given in each case will rest necessarily upon the importance, extent, seat, and nature of parts involved, as also upon the consequences produced. A superficial and slight wound is trifling; a deep wound, however slight in extent, may have occasioned persistent troubles. Wounds of the joints are always serious.

Exsections and Amputations.

§ 384. Exsections applied to the bones of the limbs, whether in their continuity or in their contiguity, are always causes for rejection and often for discharge. The same rule, for a still stronger reason, will apply to loss of limbs by amputation.

Fractures.

§ 385. Fractures of the limbs, simple, recent, or united by a small non-prominent callus, without deformity, are not a cause for rejection. But the same will not be the case when the fracture is of long standing, badly united, or has occasioned a false articulation, or again, when union has taken place with an exuberant callus, angular and voluminous, with or without shortening of the limb. All such cases afford causes for rejection or discharge.

Sprains and Luxations.

§ 386. Recent sprains are generally recovered from without serious consequences, but the possibility of consecutive disability, should lead the examining surgeon to bestow the greatest care upon the examination of those individual cases, concerning which his decision is required.

Old sprains, when accompanied by swelling, pain, and difficulty in walking, are always a cause for rejection. If the sprain is of an upper limb, its consequences are less serious, and it often justifies a favorable prognosis.

Congenital luxation, particularly of the femur, justifies the rejection of a party; the same rule does not obtain, however, when it is accidental, and properly reduced, unless it has given rise to injurious consequences, such as partial paralysis, with atrophy of the limb, which are sufficient causes of disqualification.

Old and properly reduced luxations do not justify rejection, unless they have been followed by serious consequences which interfere with the play of the articulation.

Badly reduced luxations, together with unreduced luxations, are always a disqualification for military service.

Arthritis and Hydrarthrosis.

§ 387. Arthritis, and even hydrarthrosis, when simple and recent, justify neither the rejection nor the discharge of a party, whatever may have been their origin, whether accidental or gonorrhœal, with the exception, however, of inflammation of the shoulder or hip joint, which are often serious, and demand all the attention of the surgeon. These diseases, when chronic, are, on the contrary, always causes for rejection, and sometimes for discharge. The same rule, for still stronger reasons, will apply to well-marked white swellings of the joints, complicated or not with sinuses or ulcerations.

Varices.

§ 388. Varices which are fluctuating, knotty, and livid tumors, formed by the permanent distension and elongation of the veins, may be considered as exclusively confined to the lower limbs, so rarely are they encountered in the arms. Their existence in young men, whenever they cannot be explained by any local cause or professional influence, may be referred to some obstacle to the flow of the blood, either from compression of some venous trunk by a tumor, or by some lesion in the central organs of circulation or respiration. It is therefore under this aspect that investigations should be made, and whenever the presence of varices is added to other signs, even obscure, of any of the foregoing diseases, the decision should lean towards the side of rejection. Except in such instances, no attention need be paid to scattered and superficial varices which are without importance. But when they are deep seated, and detached, in knotty clusters, extending to the thigh, and even to the groin, they must be considered a disqualification for the military service. Sometimes swelling of a lower limb is noticed, which springs from no other cause than deep-seated varices often associated with serious internal disease. Such cases justify rejection.

Among soldiers, it must not be forgotten that varices which might be troublesome when men are forced to make long and rapid marches, do not prevent them from serving in some sedentary capacity.

Abscess.

§ 389. Acute abscess occurring in the limbs, if large, diffused, and situated beneath the deep fasciæ, may occasion copious suppuration and extensive scars, and must be considered a cause for rejection. But if only superficial, and of slight extent, it would not be so.

Chronic and indurated abscess is always serious enough to constitute a disqualification.

Whitlow of the fingers is unimportant when superficial; but if deep seated, it is well to bear in mind the possible consequences which it may occasion, such as multiple and extensive incisions, deformity, stiffness, and even loss of the phalanges. In such cases rejection must follow.

Œdema of the Limbs.

§ 390. Œdema of the limbs, which is often suggestive of organic disease of the heart and kidney, may be artificially produced by the application of ligatures impeding circulation. The possibility of such things should always awaken the attention of surgeons.

Elephantiasis of the limbs when present, always constitutes a cause for rejection.

Neuralgia.—Rheumatism.

§ 391. Chronic neuralgias, like sciatica and chronic rheumatic pains, which occasion a real impediment to the discharge of a soldier's duties, are too easily feigned not to be often alleged, although young men are much less subject to them than persons of more mature age. When the pains are very intense, and have lasted for some time, they always produce an emaciation, and sensible weakness in the strength of the limbs, whose muscles, diminished in volume, become flaccid, and whose form sometimes undergoes alteration. Where no apparent symptom reveals the presence of these affections, the surgeon may draw some conclusions from the pro-

9

fession of the party and his local habits. It is well known that country people are more subject to these diseases than city people, and that there are modes of living where they are most easily contracted. In uniting these various data, and in combining and comparing them, the surgeon will nearly always be able to distinguish the real from the feigned disease. Whenever this diagnosis cannot be established, the Board of Enrolment has no other resource than proofs derived from public notoriety.

Among soldiers a powerful auxiliary will be found in those active medicines which these diseases, when real require, and which, in cases of imposture, finally succeed in wearying, or intimidating malingerers. Yet experience forces us to admit, that there are men whom the longest and most severe treatment fails to overpower. It is therefore justifiable to incline towards severity, rather than towards leniency, for fear of the contagiousness of example; but this severity should immediately cease, at the first intimation of a real impairment of health.

Gout.

§ 392. Gout is extremely rare in youth, being generally found only in old age. It is also of infrequent occurrence among soldiers and non-commissioned officers, whatever may be their age. It would, if present, constitute a disqualification for the military service.

Professional Deformity of the Hands.

§ 393. Certain manual avocations impress upon the hands modifications of more or less extent, amounting sometimes even to real deformities. It is unusual, however, to find them existing to such a degree as to require the rejection of a party; for it must not be forgotten that a change of occupation most generally suffices to diminish sensibly these alterations, or even to obliterate them entirely. The surgeon need not spend much time upon them, unless they are very strongly marked, since the manual of arms will of itself tend to restore the hand to its normal condition.

MUTILATIONS OF THE FINGERS AND TOES.

§ 394. Mutilations of the fingers and toes are a disqualification for military service, whenever they consist in any of the following lesions:

Hands.

1st. Total loss of either thumb or one of its phalanges.

2d. Total loss of the index finger of the right hand or of one of its phalanges. Total loss of the index finger of the left hand or of two of its phalanges.

3d. Total loss of any two fingers or coexisting loss of two phalanges of two fingers.

4th. Coexisting loss of one phalanx of the three last fingers.

Feet.

§ 395. 1st. Total loss of either great toe or of one of its phalanges.

2d. Total loss of two of the lesser toes.

3d. Coexisting loss of one phalanx of all the small toes.

It is particularly in relation to these mutilations that the serious question of how they occurred arises. For it is doubtless true that, both before and after admission into the army, parties do voluntarily mutilate themselves, either with cutting instruments or fire-arms. The extreme difficulty under which an examining surgeon labors, in such cases, can readily be conceived, as also how great must be the certainty of his conviction before making an allegation of fraud against any one.

The examination, made with the greatest possible care, should bear upon the antecedents of the party and all the circumstances of the accident; but, generally speaking, the question can only be solved when the mutilation is recent, and even then often gives rise to many doubts.

Permanent Flexion, or Contraction of the Fingers.

§ 396. Permanent flexion of the fingers may be either congenital or accidental, and arise from very different causes, involving the integuments, the cellular and fibrous tissues, the muscles and tendons, the nerves, and the phalanges, in their continuity or contiguity. Attention should be directed to the skin, which may be the seat of a retraction caused by cicatrices; to the muscles, and fibrous tissues, which may be shortened by loss of substance; to the nerves, whose lesion may have caused local paralysis; or to articular and bony tissues. Permanent flexion of the fingers, unless existing in a slight degree, is a disqualification for the duties of a soldier. It may be looked upon as feigned, whenever we fail to find a reason for it in the causes, or tissues, above enumerated.

Permanent Extension of the Fingers.

§ 397. The same considerations apply to well marked permanent extension of the fingers, which may affect one or more of them.

DEFORMITIES OF THE FEET.

Club-Foot.

§ 398. The extremities of the limbs present deformities known, when belonging to the feet (where they are more common than to the hands) under the designation of club-feet. Whatever may be their variety, and appreciable degree, whether *equinus*, *talus*, *varus*, or *valgus*, they constitute an evident disqualification for the military service.

A mild form of club-foot may be simulated by a false position of the foot, being either voluntary, and momentary, or permanent by reason of a faulty mode of walking. It requires no special mention.

Flat Feet.

§ 399. The bony framework of the feet is, in most persons, so constituted as to present on its inner side a hollow, whose concavity faces the ground, while its convexity forms the instep; whence it follows that, standing or walking, that portion of the sole of the foot which forms the summit of this hollow does not touch the ground. The generic term *flat feet*, is given to those who do not possess this conformation. A very important distinction must, however, be made in this connection; for at times there may be simple flatness, and again there may be flatness with deviation of the foot.* Feet that are simply flat, do not prevent marching, and are not a cause

* The deviation alluded to here consists in a twisting of the foot on its own axis, so as to bring its inner border in contact with the ground, while its outer border fails to receive its due proportion of the weight of the body.

for rejection; but flat feet with deviation, are, on the contrary, always a disqualification. If we limit ourselves, however, to an examination of the sole of the foot, and there discover no hollow, and if, finding its whole surface uniformly callous, and soiled, from contact with the ground, we reject the party, we at times run the risk of committing a great error. This false appreciation is founded upon the opinion that the difficulty of walking, under such circumstances, arises from compression of the nerves, and soft parts of those regions. Experience contradicts this assertion. Many countrymen, and more particularly mountaineers, have the soles of the feet flat, without hollow, and touching the ground through their whole extent, and yet these men are, in general, good walkers. The flat foot, with deviation, which constitutes a disqualification for the military service, consists not only in an absence of the hollow of the foot, and a flatness of its dorsum, but also in an unnatural inclination of it. In such cases the internal malleolus descends low down, and is prominent; the astragalus is inclined inwardly, and the axis of the leg does not fall directly upon the centre of the foot, whence it follows that the inner side of either ankle is prominent, and the corresponding malleoli exposed, to interfere painfully in walking, or to be bruised by contact with a rough soil. The lateral ligaments of this region are stretched, weakened, and, during protracted marches, this part being strained, suffers and becomes inflamed and swollen. None of these troubles arise when, although the surface of the feet be flat, the leg and the foot are in their natural relations. The shape of the foot in these cases often arises from the fact that the hollow is filled by the muscles of the plantar surface, which have acquired unusual size through habitual exercise. This circumstance, far from indicating any impediment to marching, proves, on the contrary, the extent of the locomotive power.

Hollow Feet.

§ 400. An opposite deformity to this, and which might be called *hollow feet*, is sometimes met with. This is characterized by a more or less extensive hollowing of the foot, with a corresponding arching of its instep. This last feature is not witnessed when the hollowing arises from traumatic lesion, with loss of substance. This deformity affords a cause for rejection, whenever it is sufficiently marked to cause an impediment in walking.

Faulty Direction of the Toes.—Sub-Luxation.

§ 401. The natural direction of the toes may be altered in different ways, and by different causes. One of them may have changed its normal place and direction, and ascended laterally, in such a way as to cross and override the one immediately adjoining; and as soon as this deviation becomes chronic, the articular surfaces themselves alter their direction, and a cure becomes next to impossible. This overriding of one or more toes, when it exists to an extreme degree, has become permanent, and yields with difficulty to mechanical pressure, interferes more or less with walking, and may, on this account, require the rejection of a party.

Some persons produce it purposely. The cheat may be discovered by noticing whether, to the cushion of the displaced toe, a corresponding hollow on the other affords a lodging place.

Walking on the Nail.

§ 402. In other cases, the first phalanx of one of the toes, and it is commonly the *third*, turns up by degrees, in such a way, as to form, with the metatarsus which sustains it, an obtuse angle approximating more or less to a right one, while at the same time the second and third toes incline themselves in an increasing flexion, so that the extremity of the toe pointing downwards rests upon the ground, when the person stands or walks. The toe is thus compressed between the upper and the sole of the shoe. This pressure causes more or less pain, the skin becomes inflamed, red, and often ulcerates on the prominent side, and walking becomes painful. Persons laboring under this infirmity, when strongly marked, cannot endure a long march, particularly when the third phalanx bends upon the second to such an extent that the toe, instead of resting upon its cushioned end (hammer-toe), rests upon the nail itself, which is then called "walking on the nail." This latter condition is an absolute disqualification. When the cushioned extremity of the toe rests upon the ground, the party can still walk, and no cause for rejection exists.

Web Fingers and Toes.

§ 403. Sometimes the fingers and toes are united by a prolongation of the skin, extending for a variable distance from their root toward their extremities, and which is designated a web. When this abnormal membrane is found between all the fingers of one hand, although it should not extend beyond the first or proximal phalangeal articulation, the party must be rejected. Two fingers alone united throughout their extent would justify a similar disposition of him, whereas, if united through a space of about an inch, disqualification would only arise if the web existed between the thumb and forefinger, or between this last and the middle one. As for the toes, with the exception of the great one, they must all be united, and throughout their whole extent in order to afford a cause for rejection. The great toe must always be free throughout its whole extent.

Subungual Exostosis.

§ 404. Subungual exostosis of the great toe, although not a serious affection, is a cause for rejection, because of the painful operation which it requires. But it would afford no cause for a discharge, unless in very exceptional cases.

Bunion.

§ 405. The tumor affecting the internal aspect of the metatarso-phalangeal articulation of the great toe, varies in importance. When it does not extend beyond the epidermis, or true skin, no attention need be paid to it; but if the fibrous tissues, the periosteum, and the bony tissues are themselves altered, which is most frequently the case, the party must be rejected. A discharge, in like manner, is called for, whenever this tumor has successfully resisted all curative treatment.

Corns.

§ 406. Corns on the feet are in general a trifling affection. Nevertheless, they may have acquired a sufficient size to interfere very sensibly with walking. Excision is only an imperfect remedy, and under very peculiar circumstances, therefore, they might afford a cause for rejection. But a discharge could only be granted under extraordinary circumstances.

Perforating Ulcer of the Foot.

§ 407. Perforating ulcer of the foot, a disease but recently known, attacks chiefly the sole of the foot, the surface of the metatarso-phalangeal articulations, the cushion of the toes, and the heels. This affection manifests itself in a thickening of the epidermis which covers an ulcerated surface, whence exudes a small quantity of viscid, colorless, and fetid matter. These ulcerations heal with difficulty and tend to increase in depth. They constitute an absolute disqualification.

Fetid Perspiration from the Hands and Feet.

§ 408. It is particularly at the points of union between the trunk and the limbs, and where the latter are in permanent contact with it, that cutaneous exhalation occurs with the most constancy and abundance. These are the chief sources of the smell which it emits. Now this odor may habitually be of so fetid a character, as to constitute a good cause for the rejection of a party. But it can be readily conceived that much caution is needed in forming a decision, for there are individuals in whom this serious inconvenience only manifests itself during exercise. They can therefore readily conceal it, or even if they disclose it, it is difficult to establish its reality. On the other hand, it is often feigned, notwithstanding the fact that when real, this odor is so entirely *sui generis*, as to be readily distinguished. It should not then be admitted as a cause for rejection until authenticated by reliable testimony, or unless it persistently showed itself after subjecting the individual to repeated washings with soap and water. Nor should it be forgotten, either, that it sometimes depends upon the avocation followed, and that consequently it may be removed by change of circumstances, such, for example, as entrance upon a soldier's life and an observance of those rules of cleanliness, to which military men are subjected.

Diseases of the Nails.

§ 409. The nails, particularly of the feet, may be the seat of a form of hypertrophy, rendering them similar to horny growths. This condition would not constitute a disqualification for the military service. unless it had acquired enormous proportions, and given evidence of being remediless.

The same rule will apply to extensive curvature of the nails, which often accompanies hypertrophy.

In-growing Nail.

§ 410. The great toe is sometimes the seat of a disease known as in-growing nail. In this state, the nail either grows in an abnormal direction, or else encroached upon by the soft parts around it, which have themselves been compressed by too tight a shoe, it burrows into the flesh beneath its lateral edge. Irritation of the parts ensues; ulcers are formed which occasion the development of soft, sometimes fungous flesh; and lancinating pains, always aggravated by walking, accompany the disorder.

In-growing nail, being susceptible of cure, does not justify rejection, unless it should exhibit an exceptional degree of severity, and be complicated with a fungous state of the surrounding flesh. It can only rarely afford a cause for discharge.

Syphilitic Affection of the Nail.

§ 411. Syphilitic ulcer of the nail, which may counterfeit in-growing nail, does not, of necessity, constitute a disqualification for the military service.

DISEASES OF THE BURSÆ MUCOSÆ AND SYNOVIAL MEMBRANES.

Hygroma.—Cysts.

§ 412. Hygroma, or dropsy of the subcutaneous bursæ mucosæ, and more particularly of that of the knee, may be sufficiently voluminous to impede walking, and thus afford a cause for rejection. If its development is only slight, it merits no attention.

The same rule applies to synovial tumors, and to the *cysts* formed in the wrist or calf of the leg. Small synovial cysts, or ganglia, such as are frequently met with on the extensor tendons of the hand, are not a disqualification for the military service, unless exceedingly volu minous.

Foreign Bodies in the Articulations.

§ 413. There are often formed within the capsular ligament of joints, hard, round, or flat bodies, mostly cartilaginous, which give rise to pain and impede the freedom of motion. These non-adherent bodies may be formed in any of the movable articulations ; but it is in the knee that they are most often found, and where they occasion consequences which are a disqualification for the duties of a soldier.

Lameness.

§ 414. Lameness may be the consequence of most of the foregoing lesions, when they are situated in the lower limbs. Hence, it may arise from congenital deformity, from obliquity of one of the sides of the pelvis, from pain, or from swelling of the limbs. Whatever its cause, unless it be an acute disease, which is known not to constitute a disqualification for the military service, it should afford a cause for rejection or discharge.

But this infirmity is often feigned, and the fraud then demands the closest attention on the part of the surgeon. It is only by a correct measurement, that we can assure ourselves of the inequality in length of the lower limbs, and consequently of the reality of the lameness ascribed to this cause.

For this purpose the subject should be laid horizontally on his back, and a comparative measurement, on both sides, be made of the space between the most prominent point of the crista ilii and the external malleolus, in passing the tape directly in front of the trochanter major.

Conclusions.

§ 415. The foregoing instructions can hardly be considered in the light of a code of absolute prescriptions. Yet the pathological indications which they describe, when judiciously combined with the results of individual examination, will generally be found sufficient to guide examining surgeons, as also to enlighten Boards of Enrolment in confirming the decisions of their medical advisers.

It is also necessary in this connection to establish, as a leading principle, the propriety of the surgeon not resting satisfied with convincing himself alone of the existence of the fact to which his attention is called, but seeking also to impart a like conviction to his colleagues in the Board. It is well, therefore, whenever possible, to sustain his opinion by a sensible, material, and evident demonstration, instead of limiting himself to a simple declaration of it. But in following this course one danger must be avoided, and that is the tendency to be captivated by the ease of explaining external affections, to the neglect of internal diseases, which are nearly always of more serious character. Boards of Enrolment are in general disposed to reject parties for visible and palpable infirmities, although often of a trifling character, while they are much more strictly disposed towards visceral lesions which they cannot perceive. It becomes the duty of the examining surgeon, under such circumstances, to unfold the great importance of these structural alterations, and to explain the consequences to which they may give rise.

In conducting the personal examination of a party, kindness, forbearance, and patience of attention to his statements should be exhibited; he should be saved from indiscreet curiosity, and proper precautions be observed to spare the becoming sensitiveness of families, on the score of hereditary diseases.

In conclusion, examining surgeons should remember the double duty they are called upon to discharge, in securing healthy recruits for the army, and in protecting the interests of the infirm. Whenever, therefore, they entertain any serious doubt of the physical capacity of an individual, they must act conscientiously, and as the law directs, by advising his rejection.

APPENDIX.

APPENDIX.

[OFFICIAL.]

PROVOST-MARSHAL GENERAL'S BUREAU.

INSTRUCTIONS FOR THE PHYSICAL EXAMINATION OF DRAFTED MEN.

I. THE duty of inspecting drafted men, and of determining whether they are fit or unfit for the military service of the country, requires the utmost impartiality, skill, and circumspection on the part of the Examining Surgeon and Board of Enrolment, for upon the manner in which this duty is performed, will depend in a very great degree the efficiency of the Army.

II. In the examination of drafted men, the Examining Surgeons will bear in mind, that the object of the Government, is to secure the services of men who are effective, able-bodied, sober, and free from disqualifying diseases.

III. The Examining Surgeons will also remember that the object of the drafted men in claiming exemption may be to escape from service by pretended, simulated, or factitious diseases, or by exaggerating or aggravating those that really exist, and that the design of substitutes frequently is, to conceal disqualifying infirmities.

IV. The examination of a drafted man by the Examining Surgeon is to be conducted in the day-time, in the presence of the Board of Enrolment, and in a room well lighted, and sufficiently large for the drafted man to walk about and exercise his limbs, which he must be required to do briskly.

V. The man is to be examined stripped.

The principal points to be ascertained are as follows:

1. Whether his limbs are well formed and sufficiently muscular; whether they are either ulcerated or extensively cicatrized; whether he has free and perfect motion of all his joints, and whether there are no varicose veins, tumors, wounds, fractures, dislocations, or sprains that would impede his marching or prevent continuous muscular exertion.

2. Whether the thumbs and fingers are complete in number, are well formed, and whether their motions are unimpaired.

3. Whether the feet are sufficiently arched to prevent the tuberosity of the scaphoid bone from touching the ground; whether the toes are complete in number, do not overlap, are not joined together, and whether the great toes are free from bunions.

4. Whether he has any inveterate and extensive disease of the skin.

5. Whether he is sufficiently intelligent; is not subject to convulsions, and whether he has received any contusion, or wound of the head that may impair his faculties.

6. Whether his hearing, vision, and speech, are good, and whether the eye and its appendages are free from disqualifying diseases.

7. Whether he has a sufficient number of teeth in good condition to masticate his food properly, and to tear his cartridge quickly and with ease. The cartridge is torn with the incisor, canine, or bicuspid teeth.

Whether his chest is ample and well formed, in due proportion to his height and with power of full expansion.

9. Whether there is any structural or serious functional disease of the heart.

10. Whether the abdomen is well formed, and not too pro-

tuberant; whether neither the liver or spleen are considerably enlarged; and whether the rectum and anus are free from disqualifying diseases.

11. Whether the spermatic cords and testes are free from diseases which would impair his efficiency, whether the testes are within the scrotum, and whether he has any rupture.

12. Whether there is any organic disease of the kidneys or bladder, or permanent stricture of the urethra.

13. Whether his physical development is good, and constitution neither naturally feeble, nor impaired by disease, habitual intemperance, nor solitary vice; whether he is free from phthisis, scrofula, and constitutional syphilis; and whether he is epileptic, imbecile, or insane.

DISEASES OR INFIRMITIES, WHICH DISQUALIFY FOR MILITARY SERVICE.

1. *Manifest imbecility* or *insanity.*

2. *Epilepsy.* For this disability, the statement of the drafted man is insufficient, and the fact must be established by the duly attested affidavit of a physician of good standing; who has attended him in a convulsion.

3. *Paralysis, general, or of one limb, or chorea*—their existence to be adequately determined.

4. *Acute or organic disease of the brain or spinal cord;* of the *heart* or *lungs;* of the *stomach* or *intestines;* of the *liver* or *spleen;* of the *kidneys* or *bladder*—sufficient to have impaired the general health, or so well marked as to leave no reasonable doubt of the man's incapacity for military service.

5. *Confirmed consumption; cancer; aneurism* of the *large arteries.*

6. *Inveterate and extensive disease of the skin,* which will necessarily impair his efficiency as a soldier.

7. *Decided feebleness of constitution*, whether naturally, or acquired.

8. *Scrofula, or constitutional syphilis*, which has resisted treatment, and seriously impaired his general health.

9. *Habitual* and *confirmed intemperance*, or *solitary vice*, in degree sufficient to have materially enfeebled the constitution.

10. *Chronic rheumatism*, unless manifested by positive change of structure, wasting of the affected limb, or puffiness or distortion of the joints, does not exempt. Impaired motion of *joints*, and *contraction* of the *limbs*, alleged to arise from rheumatism, and in which the nutrition of the limb is not manifestly impaired, are to be proved by examination, while in a state of anæsthesia, induced by ether only.

11. Pain, whether simulating headache, neuralgia in any of its forms, rheumatism, lumbago, or affections of the muscles, bones, or joints, is a symptom of disease so easily pretended, that it is not to be admitted as a cause for exemption, unless accompanied with manifest derangement of the general health, wasting of a limb, or other positive sign of disqualifying local disease.

12. *Great injuries, or diseases* of the skull, occasioning impairment of the intellectual faculties, epilepsy, or other manifest nervous or spasmodic symptoms.

13. *Total loss of sight; loss of sight of right eye; cataract; loss of crystalline lens of right eye.*

14. Other serious diseases of the eye, effecting its integrity and use, e. g., *chronic ophthalmia*, *fistula lachrymalis*, *Ptosis* (if real), *ectropion*, *entropion*, &c. *Myopia*, unless very decided, or depending upon some structural changes in the eye, is not cause for exemption.

15. *Loss of nose;* deformity of nose so great as seriously to obstruct respiration. *Ozœna*, dependant upon caries in progress.

16. *Complete deafness.* This disability must not be admitted on the mere statement of the drafted man, but must be proved by the existence of positive disease, or by other satisfactory evidence. *Purulent otorrhœa.*

17. *Caries of the superior and inferior maxillary*, of the *nasal* or *palate bones*, if in progress; *cleft palate* (bony): extensive loss of substance of the cheeks, or *salivary fistula.*

18. *Dumbness; permanent loss of voice*, not to be admitted without clear and satisfactory proof.

19. *Total loss of tongue; mutilation or partial loss of tongue*, provided the mutilation be extensive enough to interfere with the necessary use of the organ.

20. *Hypertrophy*, or *atrophy* of the *tongue*, sufficient in degree to impair speech or deglutition. *Obstinate chronic ulceration of the tongue.*

21. *Stammering*, if excessive, and confirmed; to be established by satisfactory evidence, under oath.

22. *Loss of a sufficient number of teeth*, to prevent proper mastication of food, and tearing the cartridge.

23. *Incurable deformities, or loss of part of either jaw*, hindering biting of the cartridge, or proper mastication, or greatly injuring speech: *anchylosis of lower jaw.*

24. *Tumors of the neck*, impeding respiration or deglutition: *fistula of larynx*, or *trachea; torticollis*, if of long standing and well marked.

25. *Deformity of the chest*, sufficient to impede respiration, or to prevent the carrying of arms and military equipments. *Caries of the ribs.*

26. *Deficient amplitude, and power of expansion of chest.* A man 5 feet 3 inches, (minimum standard height for the Regular Army,) should not measure less than thirty inches in circumference, immediately above the nipples, and have an expansive mobility of not less than two inches.

27. Abdomen grossly protuberant; excessive obesity; Hernia, either inguinal or femoral, ventral, umbilical, &c.

28. Artificial anus; stricture of the rectum; prolapsus ani; fistula in ano is not a positive disqualification, but may be so, if extensive, or complicated with visceral disease.

29. Old and ulcerated internal hæmorrhoids, if in degree sufficient to impair the man's efficiency. External hæmorrhoids are no cause for exemption.

30. Total loss, or nearly total loss of penis; epispadias or hypospadias, at the middle, or near the root of the penis.

31. Incurable, permanent, organic, stricture of the urethra, in which the urine is passed drop by drop, or complicated by disease of the bladder. Recent, or spasmodic stricture of the urethra does not exempt. Urinary fistula.

32. Incontinence of urine being a disease frequently feigned, and of rare occurrence, is not, of itself, a cause for exemption. Stone in the bladder, ascertained by the introduction of the metallic catheter, is a positive disqualification.

33. Loss, or complete atrophy of both testicles, from any cause; permanent retention of one or both testicles within the inguinal canal, but voluntary retraction does not exempt.

34. Confirmed, or malignant sarcocele; hydrocele, if complicated with organic diseases of the testicle. Varicocele and circocele, are not, in themselves, disqualifying.

35. Excessive anterior and posterior curvature of the spine; caries of the spine.

36. Loss of an arm, fore-arm, hand, thigh, leg, or foot.

37. Wounds, fractures, tumors, atrophy of the limb, or chronic diseases of the joints, or bones, that would impede marching, or prevent continuous muscular exertion.

38. Anchylosis, or irreducible dislocation of the shoulder, elbow, wrist, hip, knee or ankle joint.

39. Muscular or cutaneous contractions, from wounds or burns, in degree sufficient to prevent useful motion of a limb.

40. *Total loss of a thumb, loss of ungual phalanx of right thumb.*

41. *Total loss of any two fingers of same hand.*

42. *Total loss of index finger of right hand.*

43. *Loss of the first and second phalanges of the fingers of the right hand.*

44. *Permanent extension, and permanent contraction of any finger except the little finger ; all the fingers adherent or united.*

45. *Total loss of either great toe ; loss of any three toes on the same foot ; all the toes joined together.*

46. *The great toe crossing the other toes, with great prominence of the articulation of the metatarsal bone, and first phalanx of the great toe.*

47. *Overriding, or superposition of all the toes.*

48. *Permanent retraction of the last phalanx of one of the toes*, so that the free border of the nail bears upon the ground; or flexion at a right angle of the first phalanx of a toe upon a second, with anchylosis of this articulation.

49. Club-feet, *splay feet*, where the arch is so far effaced that the tuberosity of the scaphoid bone touches the ground, and the line of station runs along the whole internal border of the foot, with great prominence of the inner ankle ; but ordinary large, ill-shaped, or flat feet, do not exempt.

50. *Varicose veins of inferior extremities*, if large and numerous, having clusters of knots, and accompanied with chronic swellings or ulcerations.

51. *Chronic ulcers ; extensive, deep and adherent cicatrices of lower extremities.*

52. *Stature.* If the height of the drafted man be greater than six feet four inches, or less than five feet three inches, he is disqualified for military service. The height in all doubtful cases to be determined by accurate measurement, the recruit being made to stand erect on his bare feet, and

care being taken that he neither increases, nor lessens his stature by voluntary effort.

53. No certificate of a physician or surgeon is to be received, in support of the claims of drafted men for exemption from military service, unless the facts and statements therein set forth are affirmed, or sworn to, before a civil magistrate, competent to administer oaths.

INVALID CORPS.

GENERAL ORDERS, NO. 105.

WAR DEPARTMENT, ADJUTANT GENERAL'S OFFICE,
WASHINGTON, *April* 28, 1863.

The organization of an Invalid Corps is hereby authorized.

This Corps shall consist of Companies, and if it shall hereafter be thought best, of Battalions.

The Companies shall be made up from the following sources, viz:

First. By taking those officers and enlisted men of commands now in the field (whether actually present or temporarily absent) who, from wounds received in action or disease contracted in the line of duty, are unfit for field service, but are still capable of effective garrison duty, or such other light duty as may be required of an Invalid Corps. Regimental Commanders shall at once make out, from information received from their Medical and Company Officers, and from their own knowledge, rolls (according to the Form furnished) of the names of all the officers and enlisted men under their commands who fulfil the following conditions, viz:

1. That they are unfit for active field service on account of wounds or disease contracted in the line of duty; this fact being certified by a Medical Officer in the service, after personal examination.

2. That they are fit for garrison duty; this fact being likewise certified by the Medical Officer, as above, after personal examination.

3. That they are, in the opinion of their Commanding Officers, meritorious and deserving.

These rolls shall be certified by the Examining Surgeon, and Regimental Commander, and transmitted, through the regular channels of military correspondence, to the Provost Marshal General of the United States.

The Regimental Commander shall enter in the column of remarks, opposite each officer's name on the roll, a statement as to the general character of the officer for intelligence, industry, sobriety, and attention to duty; and all intermediate Commanders shall indorse thereon such facts as they may possess in the case, or if they have none, they shall state how far they are willing to indorse the opinion of the officer or officers making the recommendation. Similar rolls shall be forwarded from time to time, whenever the number of men fulfilling the conditions enumerated or the exigencies of the service may render it expedient.

Second. By taking those officers and enlisted men still in service and borne on the rolls, but who are absent from duty, in Hospitals or Convalescent Camps, or are otherwise under the control of Medical Officers. In these cases the Medical Officer in attendance shall prepare the rolls according to Form, entering the names of officers and men from the same Regiment on a roll by themselves, and send them, with the certificate of the Surgeon, duly signed, to the proper Regimental Commander, who will forward them, as heretofore specified, subject to the same conditions and requirements. If, in any case, the Regimental Commander shall think an officer unfit, in point of character, to continue in the service of the Invalid Corps, though disabled and certified by the Surgeon, he will state his objection in the column of remarks, and note the exception before signing the certificate. If any officer or enlisted man now in the service, but absent and beyond the reach of a Medical Officer in charge of a Hospital or Convalescent Camp, desires to enter this Corps, he will take the course indicated below for those who have been honorably discharged the service.

Third. By accepting those officers and enlisted men who have been honorably discharged on account of wounds or disease contracted in the line of duty, and who desire to re-enter the service. In the case of an officer, application for appointment must be made to the Provost Marshal General of the United States through the officer detailed as Acting Assistant Provost Marshal General of the State. No application of this kind will be considered unless the following conditions are completely fulfilled:

1. That the applicant produce the certificate of the Surgeon of the Board of Enrolment for the District in which he resides, that he is unfit for active field duty on account of wounds or disease, and is not liable to draft, but is fit for garrison duty.

2. That he furnish evidence of honorable discharge on account of wounds or disability contracted in the line of duty.

3. That he produce recommendations from the Regimental, Brigade, and Division Commanders under whom he formerly served, that he is worthy of being thus provided for and capable of returning adequate service to the Government. In case it shall be impracticable to get this last evidence, he may, having established the first two points above, satisfy the Board of Enrolment that he is deserving, and present its certificate of the fact. This evidence must all be obtained by the applicant, and must be transmitted with his application for appointment.

If there be no Acting Assistant Provost Marshal General for the State, the application may be forwarded through the Adjutant-General of the State, who is desired to indorse thereon such facts in the military history of the applicant as he may know, or as are afforded by his records, and forward the same to the Provost Marshal General of the United States. Enlisted men, honorably discharged on account of disability, desiring to re-enlist in this Corps, will present themselves to the Board of Enrolment for the District in which they reside, for examination by the Surgeon thereof, who shall examine them and report the result to the Board of Enrolment.

The Board shall then consider each case, and if the applicant is found to fulfil the conditions specified below, the Board shall give him a certificate to that effect, viz:

1. That he is unfit for service in the field.
2. That he is fit for garrison duty.
3. That he is meritorious and deserving.
4. That he was honorably discharged from the service.

The Provost Marshal for the District shall then send the application, with this certificate of the Board, to the Acting Assistant Provost Marshal General of the State, who shall procure such evidence of service and character as the records of the Company to which he belonged, on file at the Headquarters of the State, may show, and if satisfied that it is a meritorious case, and that the man is deserving, he will enlist him in accordance with such special rules as the Provost Marshal General may establish.

Medical Inspectors, Surgeons in charge of Hospitals, Military Commanders, and all others having authority to discharge, under existing laws and regulations, are forbidden to grant discharges to any men under their control who may be fit for service in the Invalid Corps.

The Provost Marshal General is charged with the execution of this order, and the troops organized under it will be under the control of his Bureau.

By order of the Secretary of War:

E. D. Townsend,
Assistant Adjutant-General.

Official.

GENERAL ORDERS, NO. 130.

WAR DEPARTMENT, ADJUTANT GENERAL'S OFFICE,
WASHINGTON, *May* 15, 1863.

In executing the provisions of General Orders, No. 105, from this Department, in regard to the selection of men for the Invalid Corps, Medical Inspectors, Surgeons in charge of Hospitals, Camps, Regiments, or of Boards of Enrolment, Military Commanders, and all others required to make the physical examination of men for the Invalid Corps, will be governed in their decisions by the following list of qualifications and disqualifications for admission into this Corps:

PHYSICAL INFIRMITIES THAT DO NOT DISQUALIFY ENLISTED MEN FOR SERVICE IN THE "INVALID CORPS."

1. Paralysis, if confined to the left upper extremity, and the man's previous occupation fit him for the duty of clerk, orderly, &c.

2. Simple hypertrophy of the heart, unaccompanied by valvular lesion; functional derangement of the stomach (dyspepsia); mild chronic diarrhœa; simple enlargement of the liver or spleen; a temporary ailment of the kidneys or bladder.

3. Chronic rheumatism, unless manifested by positive change of structure, wasting of the affected limb or puffiness or distortion of the joints.

4. Pain, unless accompanied with manifest derangement of the general health, wasting of a limb, or other positive sign of disease.

5. Myopia, unless very decided or depending upon structural change of the eye.

6. Stammering, unless excessive and confirmed.

7. Loss of teeth or unsound teeth.

8. Torticollis.

9. Reducible hernia.

10. Hemorrhoids.

11. Stricture of the urethra.

12. Incontinence of urine.

13. Loss or complete atrophy of both testicles from any cause; permanent retention of one or both testicles within the inguinal canal.

14. Varicocele and cirsocele.

15. Loss of left arm, left forearm, or left hand, if the man be qualified for duty of clerk or orderly.

16. Loss of leg or foot, provided the man have the inclination and aptitude for service in a general hospital, and is recommended for that duty by a medical officer, or if qualified for the duty of clerk or orderly.

17. Old and irreducible dislocation of shoulder and elbow in which the bones have accommodated themselves to their new relations.

18. Muscular and cutaneous contraction of left arm, provided the man may be employed as clerk, orderly, or messenger.

19. Loss of left thumb; partial loss of either thumb.

20. Loss of first and second phalanges of all the fingers of the left hand.

21. Total loss of any two fingers of the same hand.

22. Total loss of index finger of right hand.

23. Permanent extension of any finger of the right hand; permanent extension or contraction of any finger of the left hand.

24. Adherent or united fingers.

25. Loss of any toe or toes except the great toe; all the toes joined together.

26. Deformities of the toes, if not sufficient to prevent walking.

27. Large, flat, ill-shaped feet that do not come within the designation of talipes valgus.

28. Varicose veins not accompanied with ulcerations.

29. Gunshot wounds or injuries not involving loss of function.

30. None of the foregoing infirmities disqualify officers for service in the Invalid Corps.

31. The loss of the right arm does not disqualify officers or enlisted men for service in the Invalid Corps.

In all cases where the physical infirmities of officers or enlisted men come within the provisions of the above list, they will be recommended for transfer to, or enlistment in, the Invalid Corps; but no one will be admitted into this Corps, whose previous record does not show that he is meritorious and deserving, and that he has complied with the provisions of General Orders, No. 105, War Department, Adjutant General's Office, 1863, authorizing an Invalid Corps.

PHYSICAL INFIRMITIES THAT DISQUALIFY ENLISTED MEN FOR SERVICE IN THE INVALID CORPS.

1. Manifest imbecility or insanity.

2. Epilepsy, if the seizures occur more frequently than once a month, and have obviously impaired the mental faculties.

3. Paralysis or chorea.

4. Acute or organic diseases of the brain or spinal chord; of the heart or lungs; of the stomach or intestines; of the liver or spleen; of the kidneys or bladder, sufficient to have impaired the general health, or so well marked as to leave no reasonable doubt of the man's incapacity for military service.

5. Confirmed consumption; cancer; aneurism of important arteries.

6. Inveterate and extensive disease of the skin.

7. Scrofula, or constitutional syphilis, which has resisted treatment and seriously impaired the general health.

8. Habitual or confirmed intemperance, or solitary vice,

sufficient in degree to have materially enfeebled the constitution.

9. Great injuries or diseases of the skull, occasioning impairment of the intellectual faculties, epilepsy, or other serious nervous or spasmodic symptoms.

10. Total loss of sight, or other serious diseases of the eye, affecting its integrity and use.

11. Loss of nose, or deformity of nose, if sufficient seriously to obstruct respiration; ozœna, if dependent upon caries.

12. Deafness.

13. Dumbness; permanent loss of voice.

14. Total loss of tongue, partial loss, and hypertrophy or atrophy of tongue, if sufficient to make the speech unintelligible and prevent mastication or deglutition.

15. Incurable deformities of either jaw, whether congenital or produced by accident, which would prevent mastication or greatly injure the speech.

16. Tumors of the neck impeding respiration or deglutition; fistula of larynx or trachea.

17. Deformity of the chest, sufficient to impede respiration, or to prevent the carrying of arms and military equipments; caries of the ribs; gunshot wound of the lung, if complicated with fracture of a rib.

18. Artificial anus; severe stricture of the rectum.

19. Total loss, or nearly total loss, of penis; epispadia, of hypospadia, at the middle or nearer the root of penis; stone in the bladder.

20. Confirmed or malignant sarcocele; hydrocele, if complicated with organic disease of the testis.

21. Excessive anterior or posterior curvature of spine; caries of the spine; lumbar abscess.

22. Loss of a thigh.

23. Wounds, fractures, tumors, atrophy of a limb, or chronic diseases of the joints or bone that would prevent marching or any considerable muscular exertion.

24. Anchylosis, or irreducible dislocation of the shoulder, elbow, wrist, hip, knee, or ankle joint.

25. Muscular or cutaneous contractions from wounds, or burns, in degree sufficient to prevent useful motion of the right arm, or of the lower extremities.

26. With the exception of those paragraphs which refer to the total or partial loss of an extremity, the foregoing disabilities disqualify officers as well as enlisted men for service in the Invalid Corps.

In all cases where the physical infirmities of an officer or enlisted man come within the provisions of this list, or where his previous record shows that he is not entitled to be received into the Invalid Corps, he will if in service, be discharged, and if an applicant to re-enter, his application will be disapproved.

Whilst the government is most anxious to provide for and employ, to the best of their abilities, those faithful soldiers who, from wounds or the hardships of war, are no longer able to perform active duty in the field, yet it can, upon no account, permit men, undeserving or totally disabled, to re-enter its service.

Those faithful soldiers whose physical infirmities are too great to admit of their being of any use in the Invalid Corps will, nevertheless, receive the pensions and bounties provided by law.

It is further announced that no officer or enlisted man shall be entitled to or receive any pension, premium, or bounty, for enlistment, re-enlistment, or service in the Invalid Corps. They will receive all other pay and allowances now authorized by law for the U. S. Infantry, except the increased pay for re-enlistment. Claims for pensions or bounties which may be due for previous service will not be invalidated by enlistment in the Invalid Corps. But no pensions can be drawn or accrue to the benefit of any man during his service in said Corps. The officers and men will be organized into

Companies of Infantry, of the same strength as is now authorized by law for the U. S. Infantry. No organized Brigades, Regiments, Companies, or parts of Companies, will be accepted as such. Enlistments in this Corps will be for three years, unless sooner discharged.

By order of the Secretary of War.

E. D. Townsend,

Assistant Adjutant-General.

PRUSSIA.

DISEASES AND DISABILITIES

CAUSING PERMANENT UNFITNESS FOR THE MILITARY SERVICE.

1. Chronic and incurable tinea capitis.

2. Chronic plica Polonica incurable in itself, or on account of cachectic state of patient.

3. Incurable baldness of half of the scalp.

4. Deformities of the skull, particularly of the occiput, preventing the wearing of the regulation head-dress.

5. Loss of substance of the bones of the skull, caused by caries or injuries; also exostosis and encephalocele.

6. Amblyopia, caused by diseases of the nerves, maculæ of the cornea, or other organic alterations of the eye.

7. Blindness, or extensive disturbance of vision of one, or both eyes, caused by cataract, amaurosis, or other lesions of the external or internal portions of the eye.

8. Chronic inflammation of one or both eyes and eyelids.

9. Entropion or ectropion of one or both lids.

10. Lachrymal fistula, or epiphora caused by incurable diseases of the lachrymal passages.

11. Myopia, proved by changes in the eye; or if a person cannot be identified at the distance of ten feet.

12. Nyctalopia and hemeralopia.

13. Strabismus of both eyes, with disturbed vision.

14. Chronic deafness, whether partial or complete.

15. Offensive otorrhœa caused by caries or other obstinate diseases.

16. Diseases of the cavities of the nose, frontal bone, or upper jaw, with caries. Ozœna.

17. Loss of nose, or deformities, in consequence of destruction of its bones.

18. Strictures of the nasal passages impeding respiration when the mouth is closed.

19. Incurable polypi of nose or pharynx.

20. Absence of uvula.

21. Bony fissure of the palate obstructing speech.

22. Tumor or malignant ulcers of tongue or mouth ; extensive adhesions of the lips, or cheeks to the gums, causing partial closing or deformity of mouth.

23. Extensive loss of substance of the tongue or hypertrophy, obstructing speech or deglutition.

24. Dumbness.

25. Excessive stammering.

26. Old salivary fistula.

27. Total loss of all the front teeth, the eye-teeth, and first molars, even if only of one jaw.

28. Hare-lip, with bony fissure, or cancer of the lips.

29. Chronic bronchocele.

30. Extensive goitre, when slight pressure causes an impediment to respiration.

31. Abnormal development or position of the larynx with difficulty of breathing—fistula of the larynx.

32. Scrofulous or scirrhous enlargement of glands in any part.

33. Laryngeal or tracheal phthisis.

34. Stricture of œsophagus.

35. Torticollis.

36. Rickets—deafness, and deformities of thorax.

37. Chronic asthma.

38. Offensive breath caused by incurable disease of lungs.

39. Periodic hæmoptysis, hæmatemesis; or hæmaturia, caused by chronic disease of the urinary organs.

40. Fistula of the thorax, or abdomen connected with the cavity itself.

41. Deformities of the pelvis.

42. Irreducible hernia, where a truss cannot be worn.

43. Large hydrocele.

44. Cancer of testes, or sarcocele.

45. Large varicocele, painful in the upright posture.

46. Fistula in ano; fæcal fistula; artificial anus.

47. Prolapsus ani, and incontinence of fæces.

48. Large hæmorrhoidal tumors, with periodical hæmorhage and ulcerations.

49. Dysuria and enuresis.

50. Diseases caused by vesical calculi.

51. Stricture and injuries of the urethra—swelling or induration of prostate gland—incurable urinary fistula.

52. Hypospadias, with unnatural voiding of water.

53. Loss of one of the lower limbs.

54. Abnormities of size, or direction of the extremities, their atrophy or paralysis.

55. Stiffness, or loss of use, of the larger joints in consequence of scars, contractions, tumors, or anchylosis; concretions within the joint, chronic exudation, and luxation.

56. Abnormal conditions of bones preventing their use, and caused by either internal or external diseases (fractures &c.).

57. Weakness of capsular ligaments of joints occasioning frequent luxation, while discharging ordinary duties.

58. Enlarged and painful ganglia of the joints, forming adhesions with internal parts, and preventing motion.

59. Loss, stiffness, or deformity of thumb of either hand.

60. Loss of right forefinger.

61. Loss of one, two, or more fingers of either hand.

62. Stiffness, or deformity of finger, preventing its use.

63. Supernumerary fingers impeding the use of the hand.

64. Anchylosis of fingers caused by adhesion, between them.

65. Flat foot, and when the man walks on the inner margin of the foot.

66. Old ulcers frequently opening, particularly those of the feet, associated with varicose veins, infiltration of cellular tissue and bone.

67. Extensive and feeble cicatrices, following such ulcers.

68. Adherent cicatrices occasioning contractions and impeding motion.

69. Large and painful varicose veins occupying a great portion of the feet and lower extremities, and easily bursting.

70. Loss of one or both great toes, or of several other toes.

71. Abnormities in the position, or outward direction of the great toe, causing protuberances (bunions).

72. Extensive curvatures and crossing or over-riding of toes.

73. Supernumerary toes interfering with the wearing of shoes.

74. Tumors of the toes preventing the wearing of shoes.

75. Offensive and excessive perspiration (hyperydrosis) with excoriations of the feet.

76. Aneurism.

77. Caries or other diseases of the bones caused by a cachectic state.

78. Organic diseases of the heart accompanied by dyspnœa, disturbances of the circulation, palpitations, &c.

79. Scrofula, with enlargement or ulcerations of glands.

80. Impending tuberculosis suspected from malformations of the thorax.

81. Tuberculosis of lungs.

82. Empyema.

83. Extensive emphysema.

84. Internal abscesses—(suppurations or ulcerations of internal organs)—recognized by pathognomonic symptoms or their influence upon the system.

85. Phthisis.

86. Chronic dropsy, or jaundice caused by deep-seated diseases of the abdominal viscera.

87. Malignant and chronic cutaneous diseases.

88. Weakness of lungs, caused by malformations of the thorax, even without apparent inclination to tuberculosis.

89. General debility.

90. General deformity.

91. Obesity.

92. Epilepsy or other periodic convulsions.

93. Partial or general tremor.

94. Catalepsy.

95. Chronic vertigo.

96. Somnambulism.

97. Chronic gout and rheumatism.

98. Habitual drunkenness.

99. Idiocy.

100. Mental disease.

INVALID CORPS.

The Prussian Invalid Corps is recruited from the *half*-invalids of the Army, discharged on medical certificate as unfit for field-service, yet still able to perform garrison duty. The following are the official instructions for the guidance of military surgeons in determining this degree of invalidity.

SECTION XXXVII.*

OF DEGREES OF INVALIDITY, AND OF DISEASES AND INFIRMITIES CAUSING HALF-INVALIDITY.

The Surgeon will need to employ all his skill in this particular form of investigation, since the same cause, manifesting itself in different degrees, may occasion either full, or half-invalidity.

BODILY INFIRMITIES CONSTITUTING HALF-INVALIDITY.

1. Loss of substance of the bones of the skull in consequence of wounds, providing the wearing of the head-dress occasions no distress.

2. Amblyopia of a slight degree, consequent upon nervous affections, opacities of the cornea (maculæ) or other organic changes.

3. Amaurosis of left eye, the right being perfectly healthy.

4. Progressing deafness.

5. Loss of front teeth.

6. Advanced bronchocele.

7. The highest degree of bronchocele, the gland being much enlarged, without injury to respiration.

8. Varicocele which is troublesome, when no suspensory bandage is worn.

9. Small hydrocele, the patient refusing to submit to an operation, or the latter being impossible for other reasons.

10. Slight swelling, or induration of testis.

11. Chronic affections of the lungs, weakness and irritation in consequence of acute diseases, chronic catarrh of lungs or trachea, chronic hoarseness.

* For title of these instructions, see *Preface.*

12. Slight asthma.

13. Chronic diseases of the bowels, with habitual indigestion and cramps.

14. Piles, painful swellings around the anus, hæmorrhoids of the bladder.

15. Chronic muscular rheumatism.

16. Weakness of joints after wounds and luxations.

17. Weakness of limbs after fractures, with recurrent pains upon changes of weather.

18. Chronic varices, without pain.

19. Cicatrices of ulcers of the feet when they break easily in walking. Also, shortening of a leg after fracture, which can be remedied by mechanical means.

SECTION XLII.

MEDICAL CERTIFICATES FOR SOLDIERS.

The certificates of disability, or invalidity (with the name of the authority that asks for them), must be brief and exact; state the degree of invalidity, and its causes, so far as they are known to the surgeon, remembering particularly whether such invalidity was caused by wounds, immediate injuries* in the service, or arose as a simple consequence of the service, or not at all in connection with it.

* The phrase "immediate injuries received in the service" implies *accidents* occurring to soldiers, but not necessarily in war; such, for example, as are caused by explosions of powder, burns while firing salutes, bursting of guns; injuries received in drilling, falling with a horse, or from the walls of a fortress, &c., &c.

SECTION XLV.

SUPERVISION OF MEDICAL CERTIFICATES BY THE SURGEON-GENERAL OF AN ARMY CORPS.

Every certificate must be laid before the surgeon-general of an army corps, by the chief of its staff for final inspection and approval.

INDEX.

PAGE

Abdomen, Tumors of.................. 158
 Diseases of.................. 154
 Contusions of.................. 155
 Wounds of.................. 155
 Chronic Inflammation.................. 159
 Generalities of Examination..... 23
 Distension of.................. 159
Abscesses.................. 42
Abscess, of Spleen.................. 160
 Renal.................. 173
 Dorsal.................. 153
 Of Scrotum.................. 181
 Urinary..................171, 181
 Retro-Pharyngeal.................. 128
 Inguinal.................. 159
Adenitis, Inguinal.................. 159
 Lymphatic 43
Albuminuria.................. 171
Amaurosis.................. 85
 Differential Diagnosis of Blindness from, and Cataract...... 86
Aneurism, of Subclavian......... ... 137
Anorchidia.................. 183
Anæmia.................. 34
Anus and Rectum, Diseases of....... 163
 Traumatic Lesions.................. 164
 Foreign Bodies.................. 164
 Worms.................. 164
 Syphilitic Diseases of.................. 164
 Fistulas of.................. 165
 Cancer 166
Anus, Artificial.................. 157
Anchylosis, of Lower-jaw.................. 108
Angeioloceutis.................. 43
Anasarca.................. 41
Aneurism 43
Aorta, Lesions of Thoracic.................. 146
Appearance, General Bodily.................. 20
Aphonia.................. 126
Articulations, Foreign Bodies in... .. 204
Asthma 147
Astigmatism 81
Atresia 82
Atrophy of Penis.................. 179

Baldness 51
Bladder, Traumatic Lesions.................. 174
 Paralysis.................. 174
 Hypertrophy 173
 Diseases of.................. 173
 Absence, Extrophia.................. 173

PAGE

Bladder, Hydatids of.................. 175
 Fistulas of.................. 175
Blepharospasm.................. 95
Bones, Diseases of.................. 49
Breath, Fetor of 111
Bronchitis 139
Bunion.................. 201
Bursæ Mucosæ, Diseases of.................. 204

Cachexies 36
Calculi 172
 Biliary 161
 Vesical.. 174
 Urinary 171
Cancer 37
Carbuncle, dorsal 153
Catalepsy.................. 62
Cataract.................. 83
Cervical sprain 131
 Vertebræ, Diseases of.................. 131
 " Fractures of.................. 131
Chemosis.................. 90
Chest, Diseases of.................. 132
Chorea 62
Clavicle, Deformity of.................. 137
Cicatrices 40
 Of Scalp.................. 52
Coccygis, Sprain or Luxation.................. 162
Conjunctiva, Diseases of 90
 Ecchymoses of.................. 90
 Cysts and Tumors of.................. 91
Constitution, Feebleness of.................. 32
Contractions, Permanent 47
Cornea, Diseases of.................. 80
 Wounds, and Foreign Bodies in.. 80
 Ulcerations of 80
 Opacities of 80
Corns 201
Coryza, Chronic 104
Crystalline Lens, Diseases of 83
Cutaneous Diseases of Face 75
Cyanosis 146
Cystitis 175

Deafness.................. 70
Delirium Tremens.................. 63
Dementia 55
Diabetes 170
Diphtheria 128
Diplopia.................. 88

PAGE
Disqualifying Diseases, U. S. A...... 211
Prussia........................ 227
Diseases, Artificially produced 26
Dissembled... 26
Feigned 26
Constitutional 31
Sources of Indication of 32
Of Skin 38
Dropsy........................ 42
Dumbness........................ 116
Dysphagia........................ 126

Ears, Diseases of. 64
Ear, Loss of Pavilion................ 64
Atrophy and Hypertrophy 65
Polypi of...................... 66
Obliteration of Meatus 65
Foreign Bodies in............... 66
Middle, Diseases of 67
Internal, Diseases of 68
Purulent Discharges from 69
Eczema..........................38, 51
Effusions, Pleuritic 142
Emaciation... 41
Emphysema, Traumatic............. 135
Pulmonary 139
Of Scrotum.....................
Encephalon, Diseases of 54
Enchondroma ....
Endocarditis....................... 144
Epilepsy 57
Epiphora.......................... 99
Epistaxis.......................... 104
Erysipelas......................... 39
Examination, Generalities of 20
Of Malingerers, Rules for........ 30
Exanthemata, Artificially produced... 39
Exophthalmos..................... 78
Exostosis, Subungual 201
Eye, Diseases of 76
Mechanical Lesions of Ball 77
Foreign Bodies in.............. 78
Atrophy of Ball................ 78
Diseases of Internal Parts 84
Atrophy of.. 85
Hyperæmia..................... 85
Choroid congestion 86
Eyelids, Diseases of................. 94
Deformities of 94
Adhesions of................... 94
Wounds of 95
Occlusion of 97
Granulations of................. 96
Paralysis of.................... 96
Tonic contraction of............ 06

Face, Diseases of.................... 74
Cutaneous Diseases of........... 75
Fistulas of..................... 75
Ulcers of....................... 75
Mutilations of.................. 75
Facial Sinus, Diseases of............. 106
Occlusion of............. 106
Fæces, Incontinence of.............. 167
Feet, Generalities of Examination....

PAGE
Feet, Club-foot...................... 197
Flat........................... 197
Hollow 199
Mutilations of.................. 195
Feigning....... 25
Bibliography of (Note)........... 25
Fingers, Permanent Flexion of....... 196
Contraction of.. 196
Permanent Extension of.......... 196
Web............................ 200
Fistulas, of Face..................... 76
Abdominal 157
Lachrymal...................... 100
Of Rectum...................... 165
Renal.......................... 173
Salivary........................ 119
Vesical......................... 175
Forehead, Deformities and Exostosis of 74
Fractures of Skull ....

Glands, Diseases of Salivary......... 118
Glaucoma......................... 79
Goitre 121
Gout 194
Gums, Diseases of................... 112
Inflammation of................ 112
Scorbutic Condition of........... 112

Hæmatemesis....................... 160
Hæmotocele........................ 183
Hæmaturia......................... 171
Hæmoptysis........................ 141
Hæmorrhoids 166
Hands, Deformities of.... 194
Mutilations of.................. 195
Hare-lip, Accidental.............. ... 110
Heart, Narrowing of Valves.......... 145
Dilatation with Thinning........ 145
Organic Lesions of.............. 142
Displacement of................. 144
Hypertrophy of................. 144
Hemeralopia........................ 89
Hemiopia.......................... 88
Hernia 156
Of Bladder......... 175
Lumbar......................... 154
Hordeolum......................... 96
Hydrocele.......................... 183
Hydatids, of Bladder................ 175
Hypertrophy, of Liver and Spleen.... 160
Hypermetropia 88
Hypospadias 176

Icterus............................. 161
Idiocy 54
Impetigo........................... 51
Incontinence of Fæces 167
Urine 168
Invalid Corps U. S., how formed..... 217
Physical Qualifications and Disqualifications for............ 221
Invalid Corps, Prussia......... 231
Degrees of Invalidity............ 232
Medical Certificates for.......... 233

PAGE

Instructions for Examination of Drafted Men, U. S. 209
Instruments for Examination........ 19
Iris, Congenital Fissure, and Lacerations of...................... 81
Absence of...................... 81
Detachment of................. 82
Diseases of...................... 81
Loss of Color 81
Iritis.................................. 82

Jaundice.............................. 161

Keratitis.............................. 80
Kidney, Mechanical Lesions of....... 172

Lachrymal Gland, Tumefaction of.... 98
Tumor 100
Caruncle, Diseases of............ 101
Lameness............................ 204
Larynx, Diseases of.................. 125
Lesions of........................ 125
Laryngitis............................ 125
Lichen................................ 38
Limbs, Generalities of Examination.. 24
Diseases of...................... 186
Anomalies of..................... 186
Inequality of.................... 186
Incurvation...................... 187
Atrophy......................... 187
Contractions.................... 187
Supernumerary................. 189
Mechanical Lesions............. 190
Exsections and Amputations..... 190
Fractures........................ 190
Sprains and Luxations........... 190
Arthritis, Hydrarthrosis......... 191
Varices.......................... 192
Abscess.......................... 192
Œdema........................... 193
Neuralgia........................ 193
Lips, Herpetic Diseases of........... 109
Hypertrophy of................. 109
Lumbago.............................. 154
Lungs, Lesions of.................... 135
Lymphatic System, Diseases of...... 43

Mammæ, Hypertrophy.............. 137
Phlegmonous Tumor............ 138
Mammitis............................ 138
Mania................................ 55
Mastoideal Cells, Suppuration of 70
Maxillary Bones, Superior, Diseases of 106
Congenital Fissure of............ 107
Accidental Lesions.............. 107
Inferior, Diseases of............ 107
" Contraction 108
" Anchylosis of.......... 108
Medical Examiners, Duties of........ 19
Melanosis 37
Mouth, Diseases of.................. 109
Muscles, Rupture of................. 48
Myopia.............................. 87

PAGE

Nævi Materni........................ 40
Nail, Walking on the................ 200
Nails, Diseases of.................. 203
In-growing..................... 203
Syphilitic Disease of............ 203
Necrosis and Caries................. 50
Neck, Deformities of................ 120
Ulcers of....................... 120
Cicatrices...................... 120
Scrofulous Enlargements......... 120
Glandular Tumors of............ 121
Nephritis............................ 172
Nervous System, Diseases of......... 44
Neuralgia of Face 76
Neuroma............................ 48
Nose, Polypus of.................... 104
Nose, Diseases of................... 102
Deformities of.................. 102
Herpetic Affections of........... 103
Nostalgia............................ 63
Nostrils, Obliteration of............ 103
Perforation of Septum........... 103
Foreign Bodies in................ 103
Nyctalopia.......................... 90
Nystagmus.......................... 93

Obesity.............................. 41
Œdema.............................. 41
Œsophagus, Malformation of......... 129
Paralysis of.................... 129
Stricture of..................... 130
Ophthalmia 78
Orbit, Diseases of................... 91
Fractures of.................... 92
Foreign Bodies in............... 92
Tumors of....................... 92
Orchitis............................. 184
Ostitis, Sterno-costal 136
Ossification, Incomplete of Skull 53
Otitis. Acute......................... 68
Chronic......................... 68
Ozæna.............................. 104

Pannus.............................. 91
Paralysis............................ 44
Paralysis, Lead 45
From Fatty Degeneration........ 46
Traumatic....................... 46
General Progressive............. 46
Of Bladder...................... 174
Diphtheritic..................... 117
Of Eyelids...................... 96
Of Face......................... 76
Of Lips......................... 110
Of Œsophagus.................. 129
Penis, Diseases of.................. 179
Atrophy of..................... /
Loss of.........................
Pelvis, Congenital Deformities 162
Relaxation of Symphyses........ 162
Fistulas of..................... 163
Tumors of...................... 163
Pericarditis......................... 144
Pericardium, Adhesion of............ 145
Perineum, Wounds of................ 162

PAGE
Periostosis and Exostosis.......... ... 50
Peritonitis, Traumatic............ ... 155
Perspiration, Fetid of Feet.......... 202
Pharynx, Diseases of................ 127
Traumatic Lesions of............ 127
Anomalies of..... 127
Foreign Bodies in............... 127
Pharyngitis 128
Phthisis.......... 139
Phymosis, and Paraphymosis.........
Pleuritic Effusions............... ... 142
Photophobia 89
Pneumonia, Chronic................. 139
Pott's Disease...................... 152
Prostate Gland, Disease of............
Presbyopia 88
Pseudoblepsia....................... 89
Psoas Abscess...................... 154
Pterygion 91
Puncta Lachrymalia, Obliteration of.. 100
Deviation of..................... 100
Pupil, Dilatation of................ 82

Ranula............................. 119
Rectum, Procidentia of Mucous Membrane............ 167
Prolapsus of.................... 167
Rheumatism....................... 193
Ribs, Diseases and Mechanical Lesions of 136

Salivary Fistulas................... 119
Saliva, Involuntary Flow of 119
Salivary Glands, Diseases of......... 118
Enlargement and Degeneration of 118
Sclerotic, Diseases of 83
Scrofula 34
Scrotum, Wounds, &c 180
Cutaneous Diseases of....... ... 181
Scrotum, Encysted Tumors.......... 183
Fistulas of...................... 183
Elephantiasis of 183
Scurvy............................ 36
Skull, Diseases of 53
Somnambulism....... 62
Spermatic Cord, Diseases of 185
Spermatorrhœa 185
Spina Bifida............ 153
Spine, Curvatures of............. ... 148
Stammering 116
Staphyloma 81
Stature, of French Army............ 16
Stature and Weight, Minima of...... 24
Sternum, Diseases and Lesions of..... 136
Stomatitis......................... 111
Strabismus 92
Stricture, of Rectum 166
Of Urethra 177
Of Œsophagus 130
Syphilis 35

Tænia 161
Teeth, Loss of..................... 112
Congenital Absence of........... 113

PAGE
Teeth, Anomalies of................. 114
Supernumerary.... 114
Deviation and Fistulas.......... 114
Tendons, Retraction and Rupture of.. 48
Tendinous Ganglia, Affections of 48
Testicles, Diseases of............... 183
Thorax, Generalities of Examination. 22
Minimum Circumference......... 23
Deformities of...............133, 133
Wounds of...................... 134
Foreign Bodies in............... 134
Tinea Capitis.. 51
Toes, Faulty Direction of............ 199
Tongue, Diseases of................. 114
Prolapsus of.................... 115
Division and Hypertrophy....... 115
Mechanical Lesions of........... 115
Partial Loss.................... 115
Retraction 115
Adhesions...................... 115
Tonsils, Atrophy and Hypertrophy... 119
Torticollis......................... 122
Articular...................... 131
Trachea, Diseases of... 125
Tremor, Habitual.................. 47
Trichiasis....................... . 94
Tuberculosis....................... 37
Tumors, Cancroid and Fibro-Plastic.. 38
Erectile....................... 40
Of Face 75
Fatty and Encysted............ 42
Inguinal....................... 158
Lachrymal.................... 100
Of Neck... 121
Of Orbit...................... 92
Of Pelvis..................... 163
Of Scalp..................... 52
Of Skull 53
Steatomatous 40
Tympanum, Perforation of.......... 67

Ulcers............................ 39
Of Face....... 75
Of the Pharynx............... 128
Perforating of Foot............. 202
Urethra, Diseases of................ 176
Anomalies of 176
Inflammation of................ 178
Urine, Incontinence of.............. 168
Retention of... 169
Uvula, Diseases of................ 118

Varicocele.......................... 182
Varices............................ 192
Velum Palati, Diseases of............ 117
Absence, Division, Loss of Substance....................... 117
Vertebræ, Diseases of Cervical....... 131
Vertigo, Epileptic.................. 61
Vomiting at Will........ 160
Weight, Relation to Stature......... 24

Xerosis 91

NORMAN
PUBLISHING ®

Collaborators on the production of
Hints on the Preservation of Health in Armies and
Manual of Instructions for Military Surgeons:

Jill Lustig, Project Manager
Seventeenth Street Studios, Designer
Martha Nicholson Steele, Editor
Technical Publications, Electronic Page Composition
Thomson-Shore, Printer and Binder

The display and text type for the new Introduction
is Bodoni, a Postscript font from Adobe Systems.